The Health Practitioner's Guide to Climate Change

The Health Practitioner's Guide to Climate Change

Diagnosis and Cure

Edited by

*Jenny Griffiths, Mala Rao, Fiona Adshead
and Allison Thorpe*

Sponsored by the National Heart Forum and
the National Social Marketing Centre.

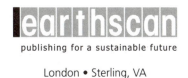

publishing for a sustainable future

London • Sterling, VA

First published by Earthscan in the UK and USA in 2009

HB ISBN: 978-1-84407-728-1
PB ISBN: 978-1-84407- 729-8
Typeset by Safehouse Creative
Cover design by Clifford Hayes

For a full list of publications please contact:

Earthscan
Dunstan House
14a St Cross St
London, EC1N 8XA, UK
Tel: +44 (0)20 7841 1930
Fax: +44 (0)20 7242 1474
Email: earthinfo@earthscan.co.uk
Web: www.earthscan.co.uk

22883 Quicksilver Drive, Sterling, VA 20166-2012, USA

Earthscan publishes in association with the International Institute for Environment
and Development

A catalogue record for this book is available from the British Library

Library of Congress Cataloging-in-Publication Data
The health practitioner's guide to climate change : diagnosis and cure / edited by
Jenny Griffiths ... [et al.].
        p. ; cm.
    Includes bibliographical references and index.
ISBN 978-1-84407-728-1 (hardback) – ISBN 978-1-84407-729-8 (pbk.)
1. Environmental health. 2. Climatic changes – Health aspects. I Griffiths, Jenny.
    [DNLM: 1. Climate. 2. Acclimatization. 3. Community Health Services. 4.
Environmental Exposure–adverse effects. 5. Public Health. 6. Risk Factors. WB 700
H4335 2009]
    RA566, H435 2009
    613'.1–dc22

2009012109

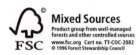

Mixed Sources
Product group from well-managed
forests and other controlled sources
www.fsc.org Cert no. TT-COC-2082
© 1996 Forest Stewardship Council

Contents

About the Editors and Authors

Editors

Jenny Griffiths

Jenny Griffiths is a former health service manager and chief executive, who now works independently. She is a non-executive director on the Board of the National Institute for Health and Clinical Excellence (NICE). She is joint coordinator of the Health and Sustainable Development Network and is the joint author, with Lindsey Stewart, of the Faculty of Public Health's *Sustaining a Healthy Future: Taking Action on Climate Change*. She was director of the Shaping the Future collaboration for specialized health promotion in the UK from 2006–2009 and has a strong interest in multidisciplinary public health workforce development.

Mala Rao

Mala Rao has been director of the first Indian Institute of Public Health, based in Hyderabad, since July 2008. Prior to this, she was head of public health workforce and capacity in the Department of Health. She published the UK Public Health Skills and Career Framework and established regional Teaching Public Health Networks across England to foster interdisciplinary teaching and collaboration. She is a former director of public health, South Essex Health Authority and former director of the Essex Public Health Network. She has taught at Cambridge, Anglia Ruskin and Essex universities and is a member of the *British Medical Journal*-initiated Climate and Health Council.

Fiona Adshead

Fiona Adshead was previously the deputy chief medical officer in the Department of Health for England and the chief government adviser on Health Inequalities. In this capacity, she was responsible for bringing together evidence from national and international sources to step up government action. She has an extensive international portfolio with close links with the World Health Organization (WHO) and the European Commission. She was previously director of public health, Camden Primary Care Trust.

Allison Thorpe

Allison is a senior research associate at Brunel University. Prior to this, she has held a number of senior public health roles whilst on secondment from the National Health Service (NHS). Most recently, these have included acting as senior policy manager at the National Social Marketing Centre, networks development manager at the Department of Health and public health lead for the NHS University. She has published widely in peer reviewed journals on public health topics.

Authors

Hugh Barton

Hugh Barton is Professor of Planning, Health and Sustainability and director of the WHO Collaborating Centre for Healthy Cities and Urban Policy at the University of the West of England, Bristol, UK. His books include *Local Environmental Auditing*, *Sustainable Communities* and *Healthy Urban Planning* (which has been translated into many European languages). His practical guides include *Sustainable Settlements* and *Shaping Neighbourhoods for Health, Sustainability and Vitality*, both collaboratively with colleagues. He is involved in teaching, advice and consultancy with a wide range of organizations.

Mike Gill

Mike is co-chair of the Climate and Health Council. He is a public health physician and was regional director of public health for the South East of England until 2006. He was the architect of the first heatwave plan for England in 2004. He is visiting professor, Faculty of Health and Medical Sciences, University of Surrey.

Marcus Grant

Marcus Grant is a landscape architect and, with a first degree in ecology, he has been involved with issues of sustainable development and health for over 20 years in both consultancy and academia. He is currently deputy director of the World Health Organization Collaborating Centre for Healthy Cities and Urban Policy at the University of the West of England, and works closely with public health practitioners in the UK.

Philip Insall

Philip joined Sustrans in 1990 from a retail background and is now Director of the charity's Active Travel programme. He leads Sustrans' input to health policy and official guidance, its programme of evidence and best practice communication, and practical physical activity promotion projects UK-wide. Philip contributes to European networks on transport, planning and health, EU policy development, UK programmes such as Foresight and the NICE public health guidance and strategic partnership between the health, transport and environment sectors.

Giovanni Leonardi

Giovanni Leonardi graduated in medicine at Bologna University. After an MSc in Environmental Epidemiology and Policy, he worked on epidemiology studies of air and water pollution and natural hazards, in several countries. He has also attempted to apply environmental epidemiology to design and evaluation of public health systems. He is Consultant Environmental Epidemiologist at the UK Health Protection Agency and Honorary Clinical Research Fellow at the London School of Hygiene and Tropical Medicine.

Felicity Liggins

After completing a Masters degree in geology at the University of Southampton, Felicity joined the Environment Agency, working initially in hydrometry before moving on to strategic planning in flood risk management. In January 2008 she joined the Met Office Hadley Centre in Exeter as Climate Change Consultant, and now helps a wide range of customers, including health practitioners, understand how weather and climate can affect their activities, both now and into the future.

Alan Maryon-Davis

Alan Maryon-Davis has over 30 years' experience in health promotion and public health at national and local level, initially as director of health sciences at the Health Education Council (later Authority) and more recently as director of public health for Southwark in south London. His main areas of interest are health inequalities, healthy lifestyles, healthy environments and the links with health policy. He is currently president of the UK Faculty of Public Health, board member for the Health Protection Agency, member of the Climate and Health Council and honorary professor in public health at Kings College London.

David Pencheon

David Pencheon is a public health doctor and is currently Director of the National Health Service (NHS) Sustainable Development Unit (England). He was previously Director of the NHS Eastern Region Public Health Observatory from 2001 to 2007. He has worked as joint Director of Public Health, a Public Health Training Programme Director in the East of England, with the NHS Research and Development programme, and in China in the early 1990s with Save the Children Fund (UK). His interests include sustainable development, climate change, information and evidence, professional and organizational development.

Lucy Reynolds

Lucy completed her PhD at Oxford University. She joined the National Social Marketing Centre in 2007, after working as a regeneration consultant based at London Bridge. She has broad project management experience and has worked with public and private sector clients, including Business Enterprise Centres and community practitioners. Her move to the NSM Centre resulted from a growing interest in health and sustainability interventions. She currently manages the Evidence and Learning programme at the Centre, with a focus on researching and disseminating social marketing evidence from the UK and beyond.

Ian Roberts

Ian Roberts is Professor of Epidemiology and Public Health at the London School of Hygiene & Tropical Medicine. His main research area is the prevention and treatment of traumatic injury. He is particularly interested in the potential for environmentally sustainable transport policies to improve health and well-being. He is coordinating editor of the Cochrane Injuries Group, an international network of individuals who prepare systematic reviews of the effectiveness of interventions in the prevention, treatment and rehabilitation of injury; and is the clinical co-ordinator of the CRASH (trauma care) trials.

Lindsey Stewart

Lindsey is Head of Policy and Communications at the Faculty of Public Health, UK. Lindsey has worked in the health sector for the past ten years. Her main areas of interest are social policy, sustainable development and climate change. Lindsey is co-author (with Jenny Griffiths) of *Sustaining a Healthy Future* – a guide to tackling climate change.

David Stone

David Stone trained as an environmental scientist, specializing in plant ecology and ecosystems processes. After several years working in biodiversity conservation he became interested in the ecology of people. His work now focuses on natural environment determination of human health, with an emphasis on positive determination and impact of changing environments. He works for Natural England as Principal Specialist in Environment and Health. He also serves on the executive committees of the UK Outdoor Health Forum, and the Brussels-based Health and Environment Alliance.

Robin Stott

Robin Stott worked for 27 years as a consultant physician in Lewisham university hospital. For much of this time he was also site dean and medical director. He has a life-long commitment to seeking to improve the economic, environmental and social circumstances that are supportive to good health. As such he has been active in the anti-nuclear movement. He has long recognized the health implications of climate change. He is a member of the London Sustainable Development Commission, and co-chair of the *British Medical Journal*-initiated Climate and Health Council.

Foreword

Climate change has a wide range of impacts with serious consequences for human society. One area in which negative impacts are already appearing is that related to human health. While a great deal of research has taken place on the geophysical impacts of climate change, unfortunately, the area of health impacts is one aspect of climate change that has not received adequate attention from researchers.

It is also entirely true that health impacts vary across the globe and, therefore, to arrive at a proper assessment, it would be necessary to evaluate these impacts on a very location-specific basis. The impacts of climate change on human health in sub-Saharan Africa, for instance, would be very different from those in the temperate regions of the northern hemisphere. However, such an assessment would have to be preceded by robust climate modelling, which would reveal the exact nature and magnitude of climate change in every region of the world. Unfortunately, in some regions this effort is largely missing, essentially because of lack of capacity and expertise as well as the lack of specific information and data that would be essential for carrying out proper modelling to assess changes in climate in the future.

It is obvious, therefore, that to assess the impacts of climate change on human health it would be necessary to mobilize a wide range of expertise and talent and the involvement of a large range of disciplines right from climate modelling capabilities to expertise on the biophysical impacts of climate change and the knowledge of health specialists. This is a field in which an organization like the World Health Organization (WHO) can play an extremely important role, but it would, of course, have to be supported by a great deal of work at the national and sub-national levels in which governments would need to provide substantial financial support and overall direction.

It is only on the basis of a detailed and thorough assessment that countries and communities can come up with appropriate adaptation measures for dealing with health impacts of climate change. At the global level, the challenge of climate change would necessarily require the sharp reduction of emissions of greenhouse gases, but at the local level societies will have to adapt to the impacts of climate change, involving the setting up of an appropriate early warning system and dissemination of knowledge with which societies can respond appropriately.

It would also be necessary for governments at the national level and local bodies to establish appropriate infrastructure for dealing with health-related climate impacts, such as adequate drainage infrastructure and facilities to ensure the elimination of stagnant water, which can lead to disease, particularly in tropical regions.

This book clearly provides a very useful overview of all the issues and elements relevant to the subject of health and climate change. This would undoubtedly be a valuable basis for creating awareness and understanding of this complex area and the means by which human society can meet the growing challenge of the impacts of climate change on human health.

R. K. Pachauri
*Director General, The Energy and Resources Institute (TERI) and Chairman,
Intergovernmental Panel on Climate Change (IPCC)*

Acknowledgements

We would like to express our very grateful thanks the National Social Marketing Centre and the National Heart Forum for their sponsorship of the book to enable the cover price to be reduced.

A book such as this is the product of ideas, information and discussion with a wide range of colleagues, all of whom believe in the utmost importance and urgency of leadership by health practitioners in preventing catastrophic climate change. We are hugely grateful to you all and thank you for your support.

In particular, Mala Rao would like to thank Harjeet Sembhi and S. Aarti Rau for all their help and support in preparing Chapter 2 on the health impacts of climate change, and Sari Kovats for reading the chapter and for providing very helpful comments and suggestions.

We are grateful to Jon Bewley at Sustrans for supplying some of the photographs.

Thank you to Ian Gray at the Chartered Institute of Environmental Health for proofreading some of the chapters and providing valuable suggestions.

We are grateful to Rob West, Alison Kuznets and Claire Lamont at Earthscan for all their support.

And finally, the editors would like to thank their long-suffering families for their patience and tolerance.

List of Acronyms and Abbreviations

AMOC	Atlantic Meridional Overturning Circulation
BERR	Business, Enterprise and Regulatory Reform
BMI	Body Mass Index
BUGA–UP	Billboard Utilising Graffitists against Unhealthy Promotions
C&C	Contraction and Convergence
CBI	Confederation of British Industry
CCDR	Canada Communicable Disease Report
CDC	Centers for Disease Control and Prevention (US)
CFCs	Chlorofluorocarbons
CHP	Combined Heat and Power
CO_2e	Equivalent carbon dioxide
COMA	Committee on Medical Aspects of Food
COPs	Conferences of the Parties
CRAGs	Carbon Rationing Action Groups
CSR	Corporate Social Responsibility
DALY	Disability-Adjusted Life Year
Defra	Department for Environment, Food and Rural Affairs
DFID	Department for International Development
DfT	Department for Transport
DH	Department of Health
EIA	Environmental Impact Assessment
EIS	Environmental Impact Statement
EPIC	European Prospective Investigation into Cancer and Nutrition
FAO	Food and Agriculture Organization
FCO	Foreign and Commonwealth Office
GAP	Global Action Plan
GDP	Gross Domestic Product
GEO	Global Environment Outlook
GHG	Greenhouse Gas
GNP	Gross National Product
GWP	Global Warming Potential
HEAL	Health and Environment Alliance

HPA	Health Protection Agency
HUDU	Healthy Urban Development Unit
IAIA	International Association for Impact Assessment
ICDDR,B	International Centre for Diarrhoeal Disease Research, Bangladesh
IPCC AR4	Intergovernmental Panel on Climate Change Assessment Report 4
ISDE	International Society of Doctors for the Environment
ISDR	International Strategy for Disaster Reduction
JNCC	Joint Nature Conservation Committee
LDF	Local Development Framework
LED	Light Emitting Diode
LSHTM	London School of Hygiene and Tropical Medicine
LSOA	Lower Level Super Output Area
LSx	London Sustainability Exchange
LULUCF	Land Use, Land Use Change and Forestry
MEA	Millennium Ecosystem Assessment
Mt	million tonnes
NACNE	National Advisory Committee on Nutrition Education
NASA	National Aeronautics and Space Administration
NGO	non-governmental organization
NHS	National Health Service
NICE	National Institute for Health and Clinical Excellence
OCHA	United Nations Office for the Coordination of Humanitarian Affairs
OECD	Organisation for Economic Co-operation and Development
PHDU	Public Health Development Unit
POMS	Perception Of Mood Score
ppmv	parts per million by volume
PPS	Planning Policy Statement
RIBA	Royal Institute of British Architects
RSS	Regional Spatial Strategies
RVF	Rift Valley Fever
SEA	Strategic Environmental Assessment
SMEs	Small and Medium Sized Enterprises
TPP	Total Process Planning
TERI	The Energy and Resources Institute

UKCIP	United Kingdom Climate Impacts Programme
UNDP	United Nations Development Programme
UNECA	United Nations Economic Commission for Africa
UNEP	United Nations Environment Programme
UNFCCC	United Nations Framework Convention on Climate Change
USAID	US Agency for International Development
UVR	Ultraviolet Radiation
VAT	Value-added Tax
WHO	World Health Organization
WMO	World Meteorological Organization
WNV	West Nile Virus
YLD	Years of life lived with disability

Introduction

Professor Sir Andy Haines

Director, London School of Hygiene and Tropical Medicine

If you think you are too small to make a difference,
try sleeping in a closed room with a mosquito.

African proverb

As Director of the London School of Hygiene and Tropical Medicine (LSHTM), Britain's national school of public health and a leading postgraduate institution worldwide for research and postgraduate education in global health, I have had the opportunity to reflect on the crucial importance of environmental factors to human health. I have also developed a personal interest (in collaboration with colleagues at the LSHTM and internationally) in studying the impacts of climate variability and change on human health and the effects of climate change mitigation strategies, including the provision of clean energy, on public health.

I welcome this important book, which shows how health practitioners and professionals can have a major role in alerting the world to the facts about climate change and in assisting governments, organizations, communities and individuals to prevent it from getting worse.

Clinicians know for example that early aggressive treatment following acute injury makes a huge difference to the patient's chances of survival: the concept of the 'golden hour'. Delay is fatal. Climate change is delivering an acute injury to humanity, which will become much worse in the future and we have already used up many precious minutes of our 'golden hour'.

Climate change appears to be more rapid, more serious and more dangerous than was thought even two or three years ago. It looks increasingly likely that the worst-case scenarios projected by the Intergovernmental Panel on Climate Change's 4th report in 2007 will be realized, or even worse, as suggested for example by the rapid melting of ice at the poles. There is an increasing risk that many of the trends will accelerate, leading to abrupt or irreversible climatic shifts. Global greenhouse gas emissions continue to increase relentlessly.

If the threats posed by climate change are serious and urgent, they are not yet impossible or hopeless. However, all we need to do to destroy the future is – nothing. To paraphrase Groucho Marx, 'Why should I care about the planet – what has the planet ever done for me?' The answer is that people are utterly dependent on it for their health and well-being, indeed their very survival. Climate change has been described as a 'silent emergency'. Failure to act decisively and substantially within the next decade will have severe social and health consequences: it is an already unfolding public health catastrophe. Health practitioners should be right at the centre of climate change strategies, providing the leadership they have undertaken in the past when there have been major injustices against humanity, as this book notes.

This book is written for health practitioners by people who are, or who work closely with, health practitioners. It is a book you can dip into or read from cover to cover. It has evidence, information, ideas and many practical examples of action. Though many of its authors are based in the UK, they have endeavoured to make the book relevant to health practitioners around the world. They want you to come away from reading it:

- being certain that climate change is real and mainly caused by humans;
- knowing why it is dangerous;
- understanding how closely it is interconnected with health and health inequalities;
- believing that the changes needed are achievable, affordable and will create a better, healthier society;
- realizing the special opportunities and responsibilities for health practitioners to lead, facilitate, influence and act;
- feeling confident to explain the issues to others who are not yet convinced and to work with them to implement low-carbon ways of living, working and delivering services;
- knowing where to turn to for more information, advice and support.

Part I, Chapters 1–4, offers information: about climate change, its impacts on health, how humanity is dependent on the natural environment and the health benefits of sustainable development and a low-carbon society.

Part II, Chapters 5–12, offers a guide on what health practitioners can do in our everyday lives, at work and in the community, how we can collectively advocate for much-needed policies at local, national and international governmental levels, and how we can adapt at least in part to the climate change that is already inevitable. It stresses throughout that health practitioners are in a truly unique position of influence and leadership in society.

The health benefits of reducing greenhouse gas emissions are considerable and a major area of research within the LSHTM. A healthier, sustainable, low-carbon lifestyle benefits the physical and mental health of individuals. There are also benefits to the health care system. Finally and most importantly, the massive global inequities in health can be reduced if we all subscribe to sustainable ways of living.

A widely accepted goal is to limit global warming to less than 2 degrees Celsius (°C) above pre-industrial temperatures, which in the UK means cutting carbon emissions by at least 80 per cent by 2050. A reduction of 80 per cent sounds daunting – but many people and organizations have already found that it is easy to cut 20 per cent or more of their carbon, and save a lot of money at the same time. If we all joined them, we would be well on the way.

The long timescales of national and international policy – 2030 or 2050 – can be demotivating, in a similar way to telling people who smoke that they might die of lung cancer in 30 years' time. But climate change is hurting people and the planet now: we need to set targets for action this year, next year, the next five years. The 21st century has been described as the 'eye of the needle' century, the narrow gate through which people must pass without their baggage. Perhaps the social change that health practitioners can lead over the coming years will contribute to a 'low-carbon Enlightenment' – an era of real breakthrough into a more sustainable way of living that will improve the health of the world's current population, whilst safeguarding the prospects for health in the future.

And our children and grandchildren will know that we tried our best – and succeeded.

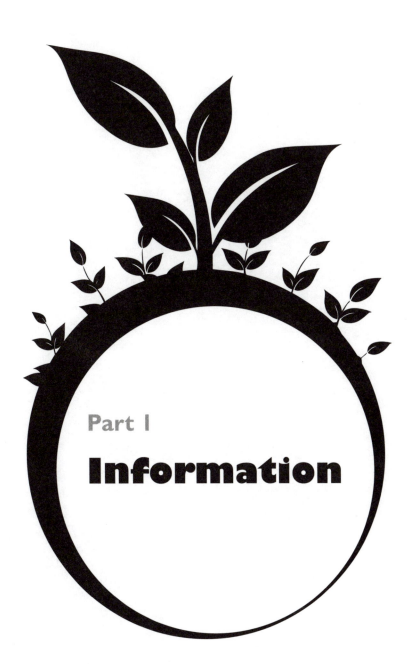

Part I

Information

1 Greenhouse Gas Emissions: The Hard Facts

Felicity Liggins

Climate change is the most severe problem that we are facing today – more serious even than the threat of terrorism.

Sir David King
(former Chief Scientific Advisor to the UK Government), 2004

Summary

Climate change is a natural phenomenon, but humankind has drastically altered the process. When we use computers to model only the natural influences on the climate, we cannot explain the rapid rise in global temperatures we have seen during the 20th century. It is only when we include the influence of our emissions of greenhouse gases into the atmosphere over the last 150 years that we can replicate the temperature rises seen in recent decades. To help to avoid unacceptably dangerous climate change in the future, many countries and regions have set targets for reducing their greenhouse gas emissions. The UK Government has set a target of an 80 per cent cut in emissions on 1990 levels by 2050 as part of the Climate Change Act of 2008. Various national and international organizations have also set themselves targets to reduce the impact they have on the climate, with the National Health Service in England aiming to reduce its greenhouse gas emissions by at least 80 per cent by 2050. This chapter concludes with some responses to frequently asked questions about climate change.

Key terms

Carbon sink: A reservoir that removes carbon dioxide from the atmosphere and provides storage over a period of time; the reservoir can be a natural sink, for example trees and oceans absorb vast quantities of carbon dioxide, or a man-made one, such as carbon capture and storage schemes.

Climate: The average weather, encompassing natural variability and extremes.

Greenhouse gas: A gas that contributes to trapping heat in the atmosphere, warming the Earth, including carbon dioxide, methane and water vapour; they are both naturally occurring and also released into the atmosphere by humankind.

Global warming: The rise in global temperature observed during the 20th century and projected to continue into the future, caused by human beings' increased emissions of greenhouse gases.

Climate change: The changes in the observed and projected climate around the world; a natural phenomenon altered due to human beings' activities; a more comprehensive term than global warming as it also includes changes to rainfall, ocean and atmosphere circulation patterns and sea level.

Adaptation: Taking action to minimize the current and expected impacts of climate change.

Mitigation: Taking action to reduce greenhouse gas emissions and enhancing natural and artificial processes that remove greenhouse gases from the atmosphere.

Global warming potential (GWP): A term indicating how much a greenhouse gas contributes to global warming when compared to the same amount of carbon dioxide over a set period of time (often 100 years); for example, the GWP of methane over 100 years is 23, meaning that 23 tonnes of CO_2 would need to be emitted to cause the same effect as 1 tonne of methane.

Equivalent carbon dioxide (CO_2e) emissions: A measure used to compare how much CO_2 would need to be emitted to cause the same effects on the climate as a particular emission of a greenhouse gas or a range of greenhouse gases, over a set period of time; it is calculated by multiplying the emissions of the greenhouse gas(es) by their appropriate global warming potentials, and is often measured in million tonnes of CO_2e ($MtCO_2$e).

Equivalent carbon dioxide (CO_2e) concentration: A measure used to compare what concentration of CO_2 would be needed to cause the same radiative forcing as a particular concentration of a greenhouse gas or a range of greenhouse gases; this is typically used to combine the effects of carbon dioxide, methane and nitrous oxide, and is measured in parts per million by volume (ppmv).

IPCC AR4: Intergovernmental Panel on Climate Change Assessment Report 4; the IPCC is a scientific intergovernmental body set up by the World Meteorological Organization and the United Nations Environment Programme to provide decision-makers and others with an objective source of information about climate change.

Radiative forcing: the effect greenhouse gases and other pollutants, either individually or combined, have on the net amount of incoming and outgoing radiation received at the tropopause, the atmospheric boundary below which all weather occurs. A net positive change in radiative forcing usually results in more warming of the atmosphere, a net negative change results in cooling.

UKCIP: United Kingdom Climate Impacts Programme; designed to provide organizations with the most up-to-date information on the nature of the climate in the future in the UK and help them adapt to its effects.

UNFCCC: United Nations Framework Convention on Climate Change; an international treaty, signed by 192 countries, concerning what might be done to mitigate and adapt to climate change.

Kyoto Protocol: An addition to the UNFCCC, providing legally binding measures to reduce greenhouse gas emissions; the gases or groups of gases covered by the Kyoto Protocol are carbon dioxide, methane, nitrous oxide, sulphur hexafluoride, hydrofluorocarbons and perfluorocarbons; by December 2008 it had been ratified by 183 parties.

How is our climate changing and are we to blame?

The Earth's climate has always varied over time. Until the 20th century, these changes were a result of natural processes. By studying lots of different resources, such as ice cores and ocean sediments, scientists can reconstruct the global climate back through the geological ages. Global average temperatures have fluctuated by as much as 9°C, with ice ages coming and going. Sea levels 86 million years ago were over 200 metres higher than they are today, whereas at the end of the last ice age 18,000 years ago they were about 120 metres lower.

Since the middle of the 19th century, increasingly detailed weather and climate measurements have been made around the world. Researchers have uncovered dramatic changes in climate since the Industrial Revolution that cannot be attributed to natural causes. During the 20th century, average global near-surface temperatures rose by over 0.7°C (IPCC, 2007). Figure 1.1 shows how temperatures have varied from 1850 to the present day. Sea levels have also risen, putting communities, large and small, at ever greater risk from coastal flooding and coastal erosion. Severe weather events such as heatwaves, floods and droughts have occurred more frequently.

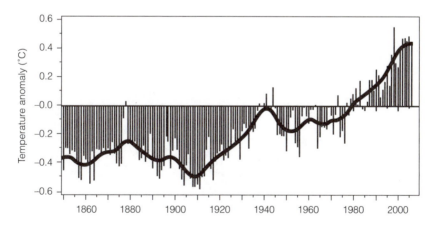

Figure 1.1 Graph showing the increase in annual average surface temperature since 1850 (with respect to 1961–1990 average surface temperature)

Source: © Met Office (2008)

Over recent years, researchers from around the world have modelled the oceans and atmosphere to see how our climate has behaved in the past, how it works today and how it might evolve in the future. A number of natural processes influence our climate. Variations in the way the Earth orbits around the sun and also the sun's output can cause changes in how much heat, in the form of solar radiation, we receive over cycles ranging in length from just decades to hundreds of thousands of years. Additionally, volcanic eruptions releasing huge amounts of dust and gas into the atmosphere can cause global temperatures to drop for several years as more of the sun's energy is reflected back out into space.

When scientists model how the climate has changed during recent decades, using just these natural phenomena, they cannot account for the rapid rise in global mean temperatures that has been observed in the last few decades, as demonstrated in Figure 1.2. The black line here represents the observed global temperatures; the grey shaded area is the range of results from a climate model. The consensus of scientists, as summarized in the IPCC AR4 (2007), is that natural causes alone are insufficient to explain many of the observed changes in climate over the last 100 years or so. It is the impact of human activities on the atmosphere and oceans, superimposed on natural variations, which has led to many of the observed changes, particularly the rising temperatures, as shown in Figure 1.3 where the observations and modelled results align.

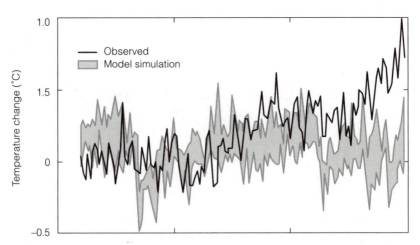

Figure 1.2 Graph showing how observed global temperature changes differ when compared to those modelled using only natural processes

Source: Stott et al (2000)

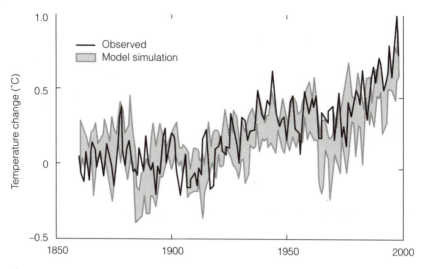

Figure 1.3 Graph showing how observed global temperature changes correspond to those modelled using natural and human-induced processes

Source: Stott et al (2000)

How do we contribute to climate change?

Without greenhouse gases like carbon dioxide (CO_2), methane and water vapour trapping the sun's heat in our atmosphere and warming our planet, Earth would be on average about 30°C cooler than the present day; uninhabitable to all but the hardiest of plants and animals. We need greenhouse gases, but recently human activities such as burning fossil fuels, the destruction of rainforests and intensive agriculture have led to substantial rises in the concentration of greenhouse gases in our atmosphere.

Over the last 10,000 years until the Industrial Revolution, CO_2 concentrations in the atmosphere remained at around 280 parts per million by volume (ppmv), after which they started to rise. By 1950, levels had increased to 300ppmv and currently atmospheric CO_2 is estimated to be around 385ppmv. A sharp rise can also be seen in many other greenhouse gases, such as methane and nitrous oxide. Although carbon dioxide is not as potent as some other gases at trapping heat, the sheer quantity of CO_2 that is emitted and the length of time that CO_2 can remain in our atmosphere (in excess of 100 years), mean that over two thirds of the projected warming during the 21st century will be due to increasing levels of CO_2 (IPCC, 2007).

It is useful to be able to look at how greenhouse gases influence the way our climate behaves when they are grouped together, rather than as individual gases. This is called the equivalent carbon dioxide (CO_2e) concentration. Today's atmosphere has a CO_2e concentration of 434ppmv when the effects of CO_2, methane, nitrous oxide and other gases controlled under the Kyoto Protocol are combined. If the cooling effect of other pollutants in the atmosphere, such as aerosols, is also included, then the CO_2e concentration falls to about 388ppmv.

So what are the projections for the 21st century climate?

Scientists use complex models, often run on supercomputers, to make projections about our future climate. However, there are always uncertainties in models; one of the most important is that we do not know how much CO_2 and other greenhouse gases might be emitted over the course of the 21st century. Other pollutants, such as aerosols, can have a significant effect on the atmosphere, often resulting in regional cooling. Predicting what pollutants might be emitted and in what concentrations is very difficult. Additionally, computer models cannot be infinitely complex or represent every interaction that may control our climate. Other uncertainties can arise from natural processes. For example, a large volcanic eruption, like that of Mount Pinatubo in the Philippines in 1991, can release huge amounts of dust and gas into the atmosphere, creating a cooling effect on the climate for a number of years. Even so, scientists can quantify some of these uncertainties, and by looking at how well the models replicate past changes in climate, they can project what may happen.

The following projections for the end of the 21st century are those presented by the Intergovernmental Panel on Climate Change in 2007 and the United Kingdom Climate Impacts Programme (2002).

Box 1.1

Worldwide projections for the end of the 21st century

- Global average annual surface temperature is expected to rise by between 1.1°C and 6.4°C (with respect to the 1980–1999 average under a range of emissions scenarios).
- Global sea level could rise by up to 60cm: local variations will result in greater rises in some regions and lower rises in others.
- Rainfall is very likely to increase in the high latitudes and many equatorial regions, while decreasing in parts of the tropics and subtropics.
- Sea ice is very likely to decrease in extent, while continental ice sheets and glaciers will continue to melt and retreat.
- Extremes of temperature, rainfall and wind are likely to increase in frequency and intensity; this could mean more floods, droughts and cyclones.

Source: IPCC (2007)

Box 1.2

European projections for the end of the 21st century

- Northern Europe may see increases in annual average surface temperature between 2.3°C and 5.3°C, but a warming of up to 8.2°C in the winter is possible.
- Southern Europe and the Mediterranean are likely to see similar increases in annual average surface temperature, but summer temperatures are likely to rise further, possibly by up to 6.5°C.
- Northern Europe is likely to experience an increase in annual rainfall totals of up to 16 per cent of the 1980–1999 average, with even greater increases projected for the winter months.
- Southern Europe and the Mediterranean may see significant decreases of up to 27 per cent in annual rainfall totals, possibly reaching decreases of 53 per cent in the summer.

Source: IPCC (2007)

Box 1.3
United Kingdom projections for the end of the 21st century

- Annual average surface temperatures are very likely to increase across the UK, particularly in the south-east of England.
- Urban areas are likely to see the greatest rises in temperature, particularly at night-time.
- Rainfall patterns will change, with summers getting drier and winters getting wetter.
- Extreme events, such as heatwaves and flooding, may occur more frequently and become more intense (summers such as the heatwave of 2003 could represent a normal summer by 2040 and a cool summer by 2060).
- Sea level rise, particularly along southern and eastern coasts, could lead to more flooding and coastal erosion.

Source: UKCIP (2002)

Could it be even worse than this?

During production of the IPCC AR4, scientists typically used four main scenarios of how greenhouse gas emissions might change over the 21st century. These scenarios were based on how population growth, economic development, energy use, technological change, society's attitudes and political leadership affect greenhouse gas emissions. Many policy-makers, particularly in the EU, regard an average global increase in surface temperature of 2°C above pre-industrial levels (1.4°C above today's average) to be the upper limit, above which climate change becomes unacceptably dangerous. Above this level, some humans and ecosystems would struggle to cope, especially if we reached the 2°C increase within a couple of decades.

With current emissions trends, climate models project a high chance of exceeding this 2°C warming over the next 100 years, and possibly as early as 2040. This means that we would need to find ways during the 21st century to adapt to increasingly difficult climate conditions in many regions – or make big reductions in our greenhouse gas emissions.

What is rapid climate change?

Alongside the warming already recorded and projected by climate models for the 21st century, there is the possibility of surprises. These could lead to regional and global climate changing on short timescales, termed 'abrupt' or 'rapid' climate change. There are a number of types of events which could cause such a shift in climate (IPCC, 2007).

Dramatic slowing or cessation of the Atlantic Meridional Overturning Circulation (AMOC)

The AMOC (part of which is popularly known as the Gulf Stream) is the process where cold, dense water at high latitudes in the northern Atlantic and Arctic oceans sinks to the bottom of the ocean, drawing up warmer surface waters from further south. These warm waters give the British Isles its more temperate climate compared to other regions on the same latitude. Several reports have suggested that this process could be disrupted by climate change, plunging the UK and northern Europe into ice-age conditions. However, the global climate models used for production of the IPCC AR4 do not project a dramatic slow down or collapse in the AMOC by the end of the 21st century. In fact, some northwards movement of the warm Atlantic waters will always take place because part of the circulation pattern is driven by the wind blowing over the ocean surface, rather than just the sinking process alone. This gives some confidence that for the time being at least, a warming of the global climate will not cause a cessation of the AMOC leading to a cooling of north-west Europe.

The impact of the carbon cycle

Presently, soil is acting as a net carbon sink, tying up CO_2 from the atmosphere as plants grow. By mid-century, however, it is expected that the increase in temperature and changes to rainfall patterns around the world will lead to increased respiration from biological activity within the soil, leading to more CO_2 being released into the atmosphere, a positive feedback process. This could be a significant driver of accelerated climate change towards the end of the 21st century. Many climate centres, including the UK's Meteorological Office Hadley Centre, are intending to model this process in order to understand what might happen.

Die-back of the Amazon rainforest

Some climate models suggest that in the future rainfall patterns over Amazonia could change, with the area receiving less rainfall. Combined with rising temperatures, this drying could lead to vegetation dying back across the forest. Alongside deforestation and wildfires, this die-back could release huge volumes of carbon into the atmosphere, accelerating climate change. The loss of the Amazon rainforest, a regional and global driver of atmospheric circulation, would also have significant impacts on the way weather, particularly in the southern hemisphere, behaves.

Other possibilities

Many scientists have produced estimates of a rise in sea level as a result of the continued melting of the West Antarctic Ice Sheet and Greenland Ice Cap. By the end of the 21st century, the highest projections show sea levels rising by about two metres. Over the next few centuries, the continued melting of ice could add a further 10.5 metres to global sea levels.

The sudden addition to the atmosphere of methane from the destabilization of methane hydrates, also known as clathrates, could cause dramatic changes to our climate. Methane hydrates are found on the deep, cold ocean floor and also, in much smaller quantities, in Arctic permafrost. As the climate and oceans warm, these clathrates could become unstable and methane could escape into the atmosphere, further accelerating climate change. This is a very active area of research.

Will population growth make climate change worse?

In 1950, the world population was just over 2.5 billion; by 2000 it had increased to well over 6 billion. At the same time, the percentage of people living in urban areas rose by two thirds to nearly 50 per cent. The 2006 Revision of World Population Prospects by the United Nations (UN, 2007) projects that by 2050 the world's population will increase from 6.7 billion today, to nearly 9.2 billion. Some estimates suggest that without population control measures, a rise in population to nearly 12 billion could be expected by 2050. Most of the projected increases will be in low-income countries, whereas the populations of high-income countries will only increase significantly as a result of migration, usually from low-income countries. The percentage of the global population aged over 60 is likely to double, again with most of this increase taking place in lower-income regions (UN, 2007).

These increases will have a significant impact when combined with climate change. In the lower-income countries where the largest rises in populations are expected, increasing demand for cheap energy and transport could increase dependence on fossil fuels. Requirements for more food could result in land being cleared and used for crops and livestock. This is a particular problem in areas such as the Amazon rainforest where trees and vegetation, helping to remove and lock away atmospheric carbon dioxide, are felled to make way for large cattle ranches and unsustainable agriculture. As temperatures and the number of people living in urban areas rise, it is likely that the demand for cooling will grow, leading to an increase in greenhouse gas emissions.

What is an ecological footprint?

The term 'ecological footprint' is concerned with how society affects the natural world. It refers to how much productive land and sea area is needed to regenerate what is consumed by humans, and also to take up the waste produced, given a particular way of living and the technology at our disposal. In effect, it measures how many planet Earths we would need if we were all to live in a particular way. The standard measure for ecological footprints is global hectares per person and, worldwide, this is estimated to be about 1.8. This idea can be applied on many scales, from the global level to country studies, to individuals working out their own ecological footprint.

For example, the Global Footprint Network estimated that in 2003 our global ecological footprint exceeded that which the Earth could regenerate by nearly one quarter, essentially saying we need about 1.25 Earths to support our current consumption and waste production habits (GFN, 2007). This equates to about 2.25 global hectares per person. On average in the UK we need about 5.5 global hectares per person, three times that which is actually available. The US's ecological footprint is much greater, nearly ten global hectares per person in 2003 (GFN, 2006a), whereas the less economically developed countries, such as China (GFN, 2006b) and India (GFN, 2006c), have considerably smaller ecological footprints of 1.6 and 0.8 global hectares per person respectively.

Ecological footprints demonstrate how current uses of natural resources are being met (or not) by the Earth's ability to regenerate them. But they do not take into account many other important sustainability measures, such as the health of a population. Predictions of how ecological footprints might change in the future are difficult as they can respond significantly to many events, such as changes in technology. However, they can help to inform decision-makers at all levels, from governments to businesses to individuals, how their activities are affecting the Earth's resources and guide them towards more sustainable ways of living.

What about carbon footprints?

Carbon footprints are similar to ecological footprints in so far as they measure the impact our activities have on the Earth. However, carbon footprints are usually measured in tonnes (or kilograms) of CO_2 equivalent (CO_2e). The measurement of a carbon footprint can be applied to many different activities. For example, a carbon footprint can measure the CO_2e released by a country over a particular year, or the CO_2e released during the manufacture, use and disposal of a product, or the CO_2e released by a family taking flights for their summer holiday.

Typically, our carbon footprints are divided into two sectors. The first is our direct footprint, which comprises emissions under our direct control. This can include CO_2e released as we burn fossil fuels to drive our vehicles, heat our homes or fly. Our indirect footprint is that CO_2e released on our behalf by the products and services we require, such as food production, goods manufacture and disposal of waste.

National and international targets for cutting emissions

On an international level, regulatory mechanisms for reducing greenhouse gas emissions have been introduced, such as the Kyoto Protocol. Also, method-ologies for compiling national greenhouse gas inventories have been defined as part of the United Nations Framework Convention on Climate Change (UNFCCC).

The UNFCCC came into force in 1994 and sets out a structure under which governments share information about greenhouse gas emissions and develop policies and initiatives to meet the challenge of climate change. Support for implementation of mitigation and adaptation measures in developing countries is a major part of the framework.

As part of the UNFCCC, those countries that have ratified the Kyoto Protocol are committed to reducing certain greenhouse gas emissions by an average of 5 per cent (compared to 1990 levels) by 2012. Not all countries have ratified the Kyoto Protocol, most notably the United States. However, many individual regions and countries have set their own, more rigorous, targets. The European Union has a target of a reduction in emissions of 20 per cent by 2020; the G8's target is 50 per cent by 2050. The UK's official UNFCCC target is 12.5 per cent, but it has gone further with the Climate Change Act of 2008 and pledged to reduce emissions by at least 26 per cent by 2020 and 80 per cent by 2050.

Large reductions in greenhouse gas emissions are likely to be needed in order to avoid reaching a time during the 21st century when a large number of people and ecosystems might struggle to cope with rising temperatures and other changes in climate.

So how do the emissions of the UK compare to other countries?

The carbon footprints of different countries vary greatly, depending on a wide variety of factors such as the size of the population, the degree of technological advancement and the consumer culture. Emissions figures are generally reported in one of two ways – either including or excluding the contribution to emissions from changing land use and forestry activities. When land is converted from one vegetation type to another, or if trees are planted or removed, greenhouse gases may either be released into or absorbed from the atmosphere, meaning the land is either acting as a sink or a source of greenhouse gases. This process, often termed 'LULUCF' (Land Use, Land Use Change and Forestry) is not included in the emissions figures presented here, enabling comparisons between countries to be made from readily available greenhouse gas data.

According to the statistics for 2006, UK emissions were about 652 million tonnes (Mt) of CO_2e, down 0.5 per cent on the previous year (Defra, 2008a).

Around 85 per cent of this was contributed by CO_2. Provisional figures for 2007 show further reductions in CO_2e of about 12 Mt (Defra, 2008b). These emissions values would meet the Kyoto Protocol target of a reduction of 12.5 per cent on 1990 emissions. However, the UK will not meet its domestic target of 20 per cent by 2010 unless emissions are further reduced.

Other countries with similar emissions to the UK during 2006 include Canada with 721 Mt CO_2e (Environment Canada, 2008), Australia with 536 Mt CO_2e (ANGGI, 2008) and France with 532 Mt CO_2e (CITEPA, 2008). Despite its investment in advanced technology, the high degree of industrialization in Germany and its dependence on producing goods for the export market, leads to higher emissions than any other European country, exceeding one billion tonnes of CO_2e in 2006 (UBA, 2008). The US tops the worldwide list of emitters, with over 7 billion tonnes of CO_2e released in 2006 (EPA, 2008).

Despite ratifying the Kyoto Protocol, some countries are not required to submit their emissions estimates to the UNFCCC and official figures are difficult to ascertain. However, estimates suggest that China is rapidly catching up with the United States in overall greenhouse gas emissions. In 2007, China emitted more carbon dioxide than the US, largely as a result of its dependence on coal for its energy supply.

Looking at total emissions per country can be misleading, particularly when decision-makers are deciding who and what they should target for emission reduction strategies. Countries with high populations, such as China, may have substantial total emissions, but their per person emission figures tell a different story. The majority of the 1,330 million inhabitants of China do not live carbon-intensive lifestyles. Estimates suggest emissions of just over 5 tonnes of CO_2e per person per year in China during 2006, which is low compared to the 23 tonnes of the United States' inhabitants and the 10 tonnes plus of the UK's inhabitants. Some of the highest emitters per person in the world live in the Middle East. The cheap fuel and energy in these oil and gas rich countries have resulted in emissions per person far exceeding even those of the US.

Since not all countries report their emissions every year, comparable up-to-date data is difficult to collate. Table 1.1 presents a summary of CO_2e emissions for the top 20 countries in 2000, along with their emissions per capita.

Table 1.1 Top 20 countries' CO_2e emissions in 2000

Country	Emissions in 2000 ($MtCO_2e$)	Emissions per capita in 2000 (tonnes of CO_2e)
United States of America	6867.9	24.3
China	4882.7	3.9
European Union (25 members)	4746.8	10.5
Russian Federation	1909.1	13
India	1606.5	1.6
Japan	1365.8	10.8
Germany	1015.7	12.4
Brazil	949.8	5.5
Canada	680.1	22.1
United Kingdom	654.9	11
Mexico	573.3	5.9
Italy	535	9.4
South Korea	524.7	11.2
France	521.4	8.9
Indonesia	502.7	2.4
Australia	495.1	25.8
Ukraine	485	9.9
South Africa	441.6	10
Iran	422.1	6.6
Spain	375.2	9.3

Source: CAIT (2008)

What is the make-up of the emissions of the UK?

As elsewhere, the greatest contribution to CO_2e in the UK is from carbon dioxide. Figure 1.4 shows the breakdown of the UK's greenhouse gas contributions. Of the UK's CO_2 emissions measured in 2006, 40 per cent were from the energy supply sector, with the remaining 60 per cent coming from emissions from road transport, businesses, the residential sector and from other sources, as shown in Figure 1.5.

When looking at the residential sector alone, over 85 per cent of the energy used in an average household goes on heating, with lighting and appliances making up the remainder. The service and manufacturing sectors use slightly less energy for heating, 68 per cent and 71 per cent respectively (BERR, 2008).

A recent study, 'Local and Regional CO_2 Emissions Estimates for 2005–2006 for the UK', provided a detailed breakdown of CO_2 emissions per person for each local authority in the country (Defra, 2008c) (see Figure 1.6). The highest emissions per person are in the rural, less populated areas. This is partly because rural areas often have poor public transport links, resulting in high levels of car usage. However, when emissions are plotted on a one-by-one square kilometre grid, as in Figure 1.7, the large towns, cities and transport infrastructure clearly stand out as high CO_2 emitters.

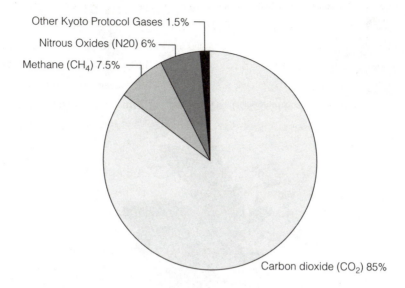

Other Kyoto Protocol Gases 1.5%

Nitrous Oxides (N20) 6%

Methane (CH_4) 7.5%

Carbon dioxide (CO_2) 85%

Figure 1.4 A breakdown of the UK's greenhouse gas emissions for 2006

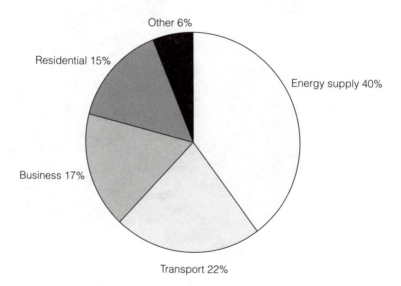

Other 6%

Residential 15%

Energy supply 40%

Business 17%

Transport 22%

Figure 1.5 A breakdown of how different sectors contribute to the UK's greenhouse gas emissions for 2006

2006 Total Emissions (tonnes Carbon Dioxide per capita)

- 4.6–6.4
- 6.5–7.5
- 7.6–8.7
- 8.8–10.5
- > 10.5

There is an equal number of Local Authorities per category

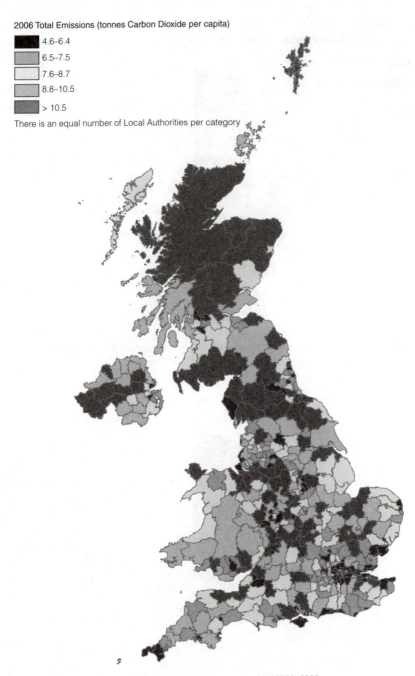

Figure 1.6 Emissions of CO_2 per person by Local Authority in 2006 (tonnes CO_2, excluding LULUCF)

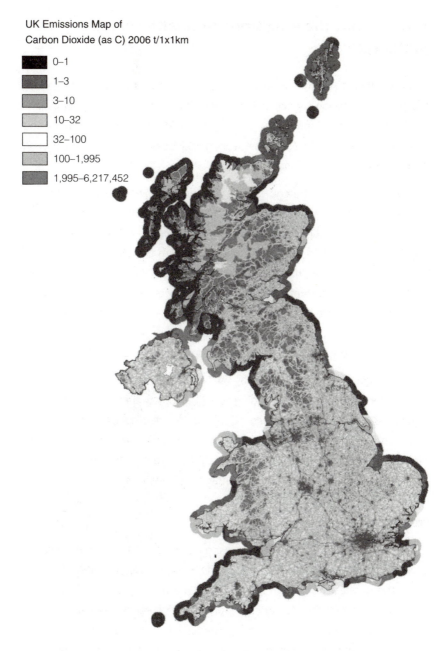

UK Emissions Map of
Carbon Dioxide (as C) 2006 t/1x1km

- 0–1
- 1–3
- 3–10
- 10–32
- 32–100
- 100–1,995
- 1,995–6,217,452

Figure 1.7 Emissions of CO_2 per km^2 for 2006 (tonnes of CO_2)

What about the emissions of health services in the UK?

Britain's National Health Service (NHS) is Europe's largest employer. Its carbon footprint is 18 million tonnes of CO_2, about 3 per cent of the UK's emissions and 30 per cent of the public sector's total (NHS, 2008). To meet domestic and international targets, the NHS must work quickly towards a major reduction in its greenhouse gas emissions.

The carbon reduction strategy, 'Saving Carbon, Improving Health', published by the NHS's Sustainable Development Unit in 2009 (NHS, 2009), proposes that all NHS organizations in England should reduce their emissions by 80 per cent by 2050, based on 1990 levels and in line with the UK's Climate Change Act. To meet this target, the NHS will have to reduce its 2007 carbon footprint by 86 per cent. Short-term interim targets have been set, the first of which is for the NHS to reduce its greenhouse gas emissions by 10 per cent (compared to 2007 levels) by 2015. Chapter 11 in Part II of this book offers information and advice on how to take action in health services.

The 18 million tonnes of emissions by the NHS can be broken down into three main sectors: procurement (including waste); building energy use, and travel (Figure 1.8). Each sector may then be split up into its respective contributors, as shown in Figures 1.9, 1.10 and 1.11. These figures were compiled for the NHS's Carbon Footprinting Report (NHS, 2008). The numbers in Figures 1.9, 1.10 and 1.11 relate back to the percentages in Figure 1.8.

Procurement

The NHS spends around £17 billion a year on goods and services, the life cycles of which contribute 11 million tonnes of CO_2 or 60 per cent of total NHS emissions. The greatest proportion of this comes from pharmaceuticals, medical equipment and instruments. Figure 1.9 provides a breakdown of the contribution from sub-sectors of procurement. Various initiatives, such as influencing contractors to the NHS to supply low-carbon products and reducing the waste produced, are underway to lower the procurement carbon footprint, but the target of an 80 per cent reduction by 2050 will require much more radical action.

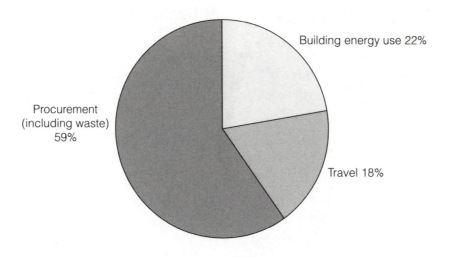

Figure 1.8 NHS CO_2 emissions in 2004: Primary sector breakdown

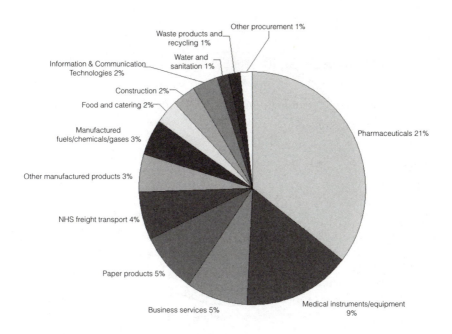

Figure 1.9 NHS CO_2 emissions in 2004: Procurement sub-sector breakdown

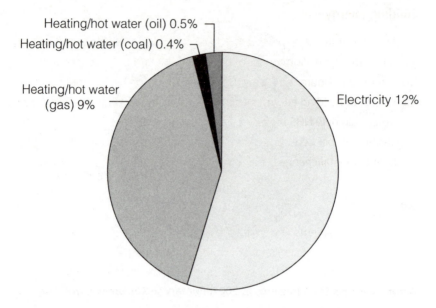

Figure 1.10 NHS CO_2 emissions in 2004: Building energy use sub-sector breakdown

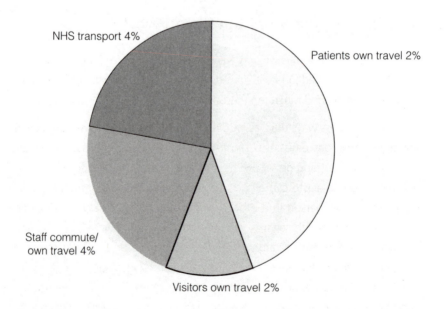

Figure 1.11 NHS CO_2 emissions in 2004: Transport sub-sector breakdown

Building energy use

The NHS currently spends over £429 million a year on electricity and heating and emits about 4 million tonnes of CO_2 as a result, around 22 per cent of total NHS emissions. Figure 1.10 provides a breakdown of the contribution from sub-sectors of building energy use. Energy efficiency initiatives and low-carbon or zero-carbon new NHS buildings are becoming widespread, but to reach the target of an 80 per cent reduction by 2050, health services will have to make more fundamental changes.

Travel

Travel by staff, patients and visitors totals 3 million tonnes of CO_2, about 18 per cent of the NHS's emissions. Figure 1.11 provides a breakdown of the contribution from sub-sectors of travel. The development of comprehensive Active Travel Plans and increased use of technology like teleconferencing are already lowering the travel carbon footprint in some health organizations, but to reach the target of 80 per cent reduction by 2050 radical strategies will be required to avoid the routine use of private cars.

So what can we do at home and work?

Some believe that the UK Government's targets to reduce our greenhouse gas emissions will be inadequate to avoid dangerous climate change, and that reductions are needed much more quickly.

There are countless ways that, as individuals and organizations, we can reduce our greenhouse gas emissions. Using our cars less; buying seasonal, locally produced food; turning down our heating thermostats and reducing, reusing and recycling our waste can all help to shrink that average of 10 tonnes of CO_2e emitted per person in the UK. As Europe's biggest employer, the NHS, along with other health services, should lead the way in the UK, Europe and the world by meeting its targets to reduce emissions and helping to avoid dangerous climate change. For more information and ideas on how you, your family, your friends, your community, your colleagues and your organization can get our collective carbon emissions under control, please read Part II of this book.

Myth-busting

Why bother reducing the UK's emissions? Aren't China and India the real problem?

It is true that the developing countries, including China and India, are rapidly increasing their greenhouse gas emissions. Estimates suggest that India and China combined currently contribute about one quarter of global carbon dioxide emissions and by 2030 this figure could reach 34 per cent (EIA, 2008).

However, this does not mean that the UK and other developed countries should not reduce their own greenhouse gas emissions. Climate change is a global problem and requires action from every citizen, every organization and every country. If we are to avoid dangerous climate change that will make life very difficult indeed for our children and grandchildren, we must all aim to reduce our greenhouse gas emissions to below 2 tonnes per person. It can also be argued that high-income countries have a moral responsibility to lead the way to a low-carbon future, because we were the first to industrialize in the 19th century, burning the large quantities of fossil fuels that are a major contributor to the changes in climate already recorded and those projected for the future. Climate change is the result of the development of the richer nations around the world, including the UK and USA, not those countries now seeking to increase their prosperity and well-being. And whilst climate change is already affecting people living and working in the UK, it is the less economically developed countries that are likely to suffer the greatest effects and may be less able to adapt to the impacts of a warming climate that are described in Chapter 2. The UK and other developed nations can lead the way in using education, new technology and stringent targets.

Hasn't there always been climate change? Didn't the Thames freeze over? Didn't the Romans have vineyards in England?

Yes, the climate is always changing. During the 17th and 18th centuries, and into the 19th, the Thames froze over on a number of occasions. The stability of the ice was such that people took to skating and curling and 'frost fairs' were held in London. The exact causes behind this cool period, often known as the Little Ice Age, are still debated. However, nearly all theories propose natural phenomena as the reason, such as decreased solar output and increased volcanic activity. Likewise, the warm period during which the Romans established their vineyards can be attributed to natural processes. As discussed earlier in the chapter, climate models include nearly all natural phenomena that can cause both a warming and a cooling of the global climate. Yet they are still projecting that the greenhouse gases released over the last 150 years or so, and those that might be emitted in the future, will significantly affect our climate in coming years.

Can't we solve the problem with nuclear power?

Generation of electricity using nuclear power results in negligible quantities of greenhouse gases being emitted into the atmosphere, and some countries have decided to increase the amount of electricity generated this way to help meet their national and international emissions targets. However, there is considerable public concern regarding the long-term safe disposal of the radioactive waste created by nuclear power. Nuclear power stations are expensive to build and can take years to commission. Some views of the future see the use of nuclear power alongside other low-carbon forms of energy generation, such as carbon capture and storage schemes and more use of renewables, such as solar and wind power. There are major climatic advantages to be had by increasing our energy efficiency and reducing consumption now, as well as in the future.

Surely we will develop the technology needed?

Studies have shown that we need to start reducing our greenhouse gas emissions *now*. New technologies *are* needed to ensure that in the future renewable forms of energy are utilized to their full extent and that emissions from fossil fuels are as 'clean' as possible. However, as the global population grows and the demand for energy, goods and services increases we cannot afford to wait to see what new technology develops. If we do not begin to reduce our emissions within the next decade the effects of climate change are likely to outweigh any benefits that technology implemented in the middle of the 21st century could bring.

How about planting trees to offset my emissions?

Many schemes encourage people to offset their greenhouse gas emissions, particularly carbon dioxide, by planting trees. In theory, this is a good idea as the trees absorb CO_2 from the atmosphere and lock it away for a long time, or at least until the tree is either burned, felled or dies (and trees have other benefits – see Chapter 9). However, the rate at which we are currently emitting CO_2 cannot be met by planting trees. Studies have also shown that at higher latitudes forests actually help to warm the climate. Grasslands, crops, or those areas of tundra usually covered by snow act as reflectors and help to cool the climate, but if these areas become forested then the warming effect of the dark leaves absorbing the sun's energy can surpass the cooling contribution of atmospheric CO_2 absorption. Afforestation is only really effective in cooling the climate in tropical regions, where the high evapotranspiration rates of trees increase cloud formation above the forests and block solar radiation from reaching the Earth's surface.

References

ANGGI (2008) 'Australian National Greenhouse Gas Inventory, 2006', available at www.climatechange.gov.au/inventory/2006/index.html (accessed 8 October 2008)

BERR (2008) 'Energy Trends – September 2008', available at www.berr.gov.uk/whatwedo/energy/statistics/publications/trends/index.html (accessed 9 October 2008)

CAIT (2008) 'Yearly emissions', Climate Analysis Indicators Tool (CAIT) Version 5.0, World Resources Institute

CITEPA (2008) 'Air Emissions – Annual National Data', available at www.citepa.org/emissions/nationale/Ges/ges_prg_en.htm (accessed 8 October 2008)

Defra (2008a) 'Statistical Release: UK Climate Change Sustainable Development Indicator: 2006 Greenhouse Gas Emissions, Final Figures', available at www.defra.gov.uk/news/2008/080131a.htm (accessed 8 October 2008)

Defra (2008b) 'Statistical Release: UK Climate Change Sustainable Development Indicator: 2006 Greenhouse Gas Emissions, Provisional Figures', available at www.defra.gov.uk/news/2008/080327a.htm (accessed 8 October 2008)

Defra (2008c) 'Local and Regional CO_2 Emissions Estimates for 2005–2006 for the UK', available at www.defra.gov.uk/environment/statistics/globatmos/galocalghg.htm (accessed 8 October 2008)

EIA (2008) 'International Energy Outlook', Chapter 7: Energy Related Carbon Dioxide Emissions, available at www.eia.doe.gov/oiaf/ieo/emissions.html (accessed 7 October 2008)

Environment Canada (2008) 'Canada's 2006 Greenhouse Gas Inventory – A Summary of Trends', available at www.ec.gc.ca/pdb/ghg/inventory_report/2006/som-sum_eng.cfm (accessed 8 October 2008)

EPA (2008) 'U.S. Greenhouse Gas Inventory Reports Inventory of US Greenhouse Gas Emissions and Sinks Inventory: 1990–2006', USEPA #430-R-08-005, available at www.epa.gov/climatechange/emissions/usinventoryreport.html (accessed 8 October 2008)

GFN (2006a) 'Global Footprint Network, United States of America's Footprint, 1961–2003', available at www.footprintnetwork.org/webgraph/graphpage.php?country=usa (accessed 9 October 2008)

GFN (2006b) 'Global Footprint Network, China's Footprint, 1961–2003', available at www.footprintnetwork.org/webgraph/graphpage.php?country=china (accessed 9 October 2008)

GFN (2006c) 'Global Footprint Network, India's Footprint, 1961–2003', available at www.footprintnetwork.org/webgraph/graphpage.php?country=india (accessed 9 October 2008)

GFN (2007) 'Global Footprint Network, Humanity's Footprint, 1961–2003', available at www.footprintnetwork.org/gfn_sub.php?content=global_footprint (accessed 9 October 2008)

IPCC (2007) 'Climate Change 2007: The Physical Science Basis. Contribution of Working Group I to the Fourth Assessment Report of the Intergovernmental Panel on Climate Change', Solomon, S., Qin, D., Manning, M., Chen, Z., Marquis, M., Averyt, K.B., Tignor, M. and Miller, H.L. (eds) Cambridge University Press, Cambridge, United Kingdom and New York, USA

NHS (2008) 'NHS England Carbon Emissions Carbon Footprinting Report', available at www.sdu.nhs.uk/page.php?area_id=7 (accessed 8 October 2008)

NHS (2009) 'Saving Carbon, Improving Health', Sustainable Development Unit, available at www.sdu.nhs.uk/page.php?page_id=94 (accessed 28 January 2009)

Stott, P.A., Tett, S.F.B., Jones, G.S., Allen, M.R., Mitchell, J.F.B. and Jenkins, G.J. (2000) 'External control of 20th century temperature by natural and anthropogenic forcings', *Science*, vol 290, issue 5499, pp2133–2137

UBA (2008) 'Umweltbundesamt: National Inventory Report for the German Greenhouse Gas Inventory 1990 – 2006', available at www.umweltbundesamt. de/uba-info-medien/mysql_medien.php?anfrage=Kennummer&Suchwort=3481 (accessed 8 October 2008)

UKCIP (2002) Hulme, M., Jenkins, G.J., Lu, X., Turnpenny, J.R., Mitchell, T.D., Jones, R.G., Lowe, J., Murphy, J.M., Hassell, D., Boorman, P., McDonald, R. and Hill, S. 'Climate Change Scenarios for the United Kingdom: The UKCIP02 Scientific Report', Tyndall Centre for Climate Change Research, School of Environmental Sciences, University of East Anglia, Norwich

UN (2007) 'World Population Prospects: The 2006 Revision', available at www. un.org/esa/population/publications/wpp2006/wpp2006.htm (accessed 25 September 2008)

2 Climate Change is Deadly: The Health Impacts of Climate Change

Mala Rao

The earth has enough resources to meet people's needs but will never have enough to satisfy people's greed.

Mahatma Gandhi

Summary

Climate change is a serious threat to the health of populations. A temperature rise of 2°C may have a catastrophic impact on health.

Climate change has already claimed many lives worldwide and its impact on human health is increasing as it continues unabated. There are substantial inequalities in the burden of disease resulting from climate change within and between countries, with socio-economically deprived communities facing disproportionately higher levels of ill health despite being least likely to have contributed to it.

The potential future consequences of climate change and the coping strategies needed to address it are being explored by scientists worldwide, through the development of scenarios and projections. Climate change affects health through direct and also complex indirect mechanisms. Extreme weather events can result in deaths, physical and mental illness and injury. Global warming may affect the distribution of vector-borne and diarrhoeal and other infectious diseases. It may also affect health by increasing air pollution and exposure to ultraviolet radiation. Increases in temperature and altered rainfall patterns can result in drought, leading to food and water shortage and severe malnutrition. The displacement of populations searching for food and water may precipitate conflicts. Of course, not all health impacts of climate change are negative. Warming may result in fewer cold-related deaths and a reduction in the risk of some vector-borne diseases in parts of the world where the climate becomes hostile to their transmission. But the scientific community agrees that the balance of projected health impacts is likely to be overwhelmingly negative.

Key terms

Food security: Food security refers to the availability of food and one's access to it; a household is considered food secure when its occupants do not live in hunger or fear of starvation.

Vector-borne disease: A vector-borne disease is one in which pathogens such as viruses or bacteria are transmitted from an infected individual to another by arthropods such as mosquitoes and ticks, usually through a bite; sometimes other animals serve as intermediary hosts.

Troposphere: The troposphere is the lowest portion of the Earth's atmosphere; it extends to between 10 and 18 kilometres above the Earth's surface.

Stratosphere: The stratosphere is the second major layer of the Earth's atmosphere, just above the troposphere; it is situated between about 10 and 50 kilometres above the Earth's surface; the stratosphere protects life on Earth from the sun's harmful ultraviolet rays.

Global distribution of current impacts of climate change

The health of the world's population has, in general, shown a remarkable improvement over the past century. Average life expectancy at birth has increased worldwide. However, this overall improvement masks considerable inequalities within and between countries (CSDH, 2008). In parts of Africa, life expectancy has fallen in recent decades largely because of AIDS and child mortality is higher now than about 20 years ago (UNDP, 2005). The burden of non-communicable diseases, such as heart disease and diabetes, now accounts for nearly half of the global burden of disease (HM Government, 2008, p103). Not only is this burden high in the developed world, but is growing fastest in low- and middle-income countries, already struggling to address the continuing challenge of communicable diseases such as malaria and diarrhoeal disease, which are far from being eliminated.

Added to all this is the evidence that climate change is already having a discernable influence on the global burden of disease (Haines et al, 2006) and particularly on the health of the most vulnerable in society – the young, the elderly and the poor – and is projected to have even greater impacts in the future. Many other factors such as the growth in population, rapid urbanization and land use changes also have serious implications for health and these changes could, in some circumstances, interact with climate change to magnify its impacts (Haines et al, 2006; see also Chapter 3).

'If climate change progresses unhindered, South Asia is expected to bear the brunt of global warming', warns a 2008 Oxfam report on the management of natural disasters in South Asia (Oxfam, 2008, p13). This is confirmed by a

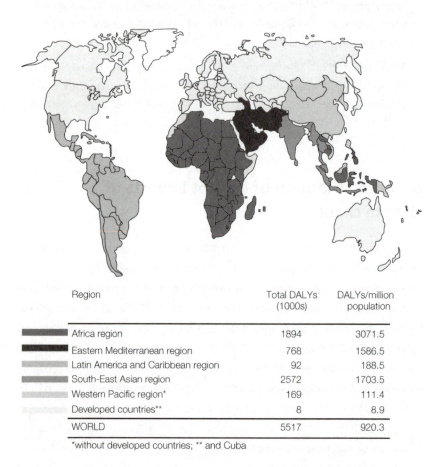

Region	Total DALYs (1000s)	DALYs/million population
Africa region	1894	3071.5
Eastern Mediterranean region	768	1586.5
Latin America and Caribbean region	92	188.5
South-East Asian region	2572	1703.5
Western Pacific region*	169	111.4
Developed countries**	8	8.9
WORLD	5517	920.3

*without developed countries; ** and Cuba

Figure 2.1 Estimated impacts of climate change in 2000 by region

Source: WHO, 2003. 'How much disease would climate change cause?' Figure 7.1. www.who.int/globalchange/climate/summary/en/index6.html (accessed 11 February 2009)

World Health Organization project (WHO, 2003) estimating the global burden of disease attributable to climate change. The analyses included only those health impacts that were underpinned by the strongest evidence – food-and-water-borne disease, vector-borne disease, fatal injuries resulting from natural disasters and the risk of malnutrition – and is therefore likely to be an underestimate of the true burden of climate change on health. The Disability-Adjusted Life Year (DALY), which is the sum of years of life lost due to premature death and years of life lived with disability (YLD), was assessed (Figure 2.1).

The African region had the greatest disease burden from climate change per million population in 2000. The severe *overall* health impact on the South-east Asia region is likely to be due to its substantially higher population density, compounding the direct effects of climate chaos such as floods and drought as illustrated by the picture (Figure 2.2).

Furthermore, social inequalities shaped by poverty and exclusion heighten the vulnerability of populations already at greatest risk of paying the price

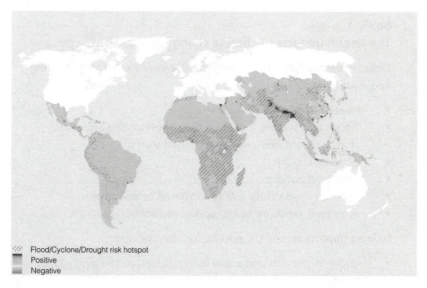

/// Flood/Cyclone/Drought risk hotspot
     Positive
     Negative

Figure 2.2 A world map showing floods, cyclone and drought hazard hotspots and population density

Source: Map reproduced courtesy of CARE/UNOCHA/Maplecroft from the joint study entitled Humanitarian Implications of Climate Change: Mapping Emerging Trends and Risk Hotspots', first published August 2008. Available at www.careclimatechange.org/files/map_all_hazards_popdensity_change_world.jpg

of climate chaos (McMichael et al, 2008) and impede their ability to recover from successive and increasingly frequent disasters. Overall, Africa's energy consumption per capita remains low (see Chapter 1) and hence its contribution to global climate change is minimal (UNECA, 2006). But the irony is that Africa is the continent most vulnerable to the impacts of projected changes because widespread poverty limits its ability to adapt (IPCC, 2001).

So what are the health impacts of climate change?

This chapter summarizes the findings of a number of studies undertaken to investigate the health impacts of climate change. The European Union has concluded that global mean temperature change should not exceed 2°C above pre-industrial levels (Spratt and Sutton, 2008), widely recognized as the limit beyond which the risks of the worst effects may occur. Consequently, research conclusions are based broadly on the assumption of warming not exceeding

Box 2.1
The health impacts of climate change in the UK

Direct impacts within the UK may include increased deaths, disease and injury due to:

- heatwaves;
- floods and storms, including the risks from sewage and chemical contamination and mental stress;
- poor air quality;
- increased pollens;
- reduced food safety due to increased temperatures;
- increased exposure to ultraviolet radiation.

Indirect impacts on the UK population may include:

- widening health and social inequalities due to rising global food prices;
- increased risks from vector-borne and other infectious diseases in other parts of the world;
- risks due to extreme weather events and climate change conflicts in other parts of the world.

that target. The human consequences of temperatures rising above this cap are largely unknown but potentially catastrophic.

The contribution of Working Group II to the Fourth Assessment Report of the Intergovernmental Panel on Climate Change (IPCC), published in 2007, includes the most authoritative and exhaustive review of the evidence to date of the health impacts of climate change (Confalonieri et al, 2007). The report indicates that climate change is already having both positive and negative effects on health in different parts of the world (IPCC, 2007). Temperature increases are occurring across all continents. Temperate countries are witnessing a decrease in cold days and nights and, therefore, some benefits such as a decline in deaths from exposure to cold. The IPCC nevertheless projects an overwhelmingly negative balance as illustrated by its figure of selected global health impacts reproduced below (Figure 2.3). Overall, the benefits will be

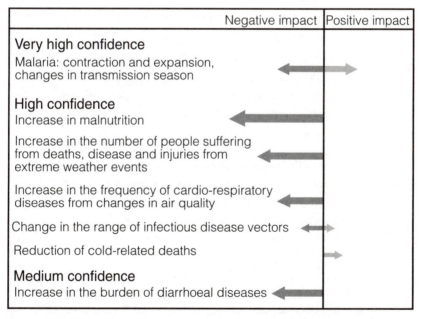

Figure 2.3 Direction and magnitude of selected health impacts of climate change

Source: Climate Change 2007: Impacts, Adaptation and Vulnerability. Working Group II. Contribution to the Fourth Assessment Report of the Intergovernmental Panel on Climate Change. Figure 8.3. Cambridge University Press

outweighed by the adverse health impacts especially in developing countries, and even within countries the balance of positive and negative impacts may change over time (IPCC, 2007).

The effects of heatwaves

Heatwaves have become more frequent worldwide and have been associated with a marked short-term increase in mortality, as confirmed by research in North America, Europe and Asia. Urban centres may be particularly affected because of the urban heat island effect, with temperatures being higher than in surrounding suburban or rural areas (Haines et al, 2006). In the summer of 2003, Europe suffered a heatwave causing an estimated 35,000 extra deaths (Bhattacharya, 2003). Nearly 15,000 of these were in France, with many deaths attributed directly to the effects of heat, such as heat stroke, hyperthermia and dehydration (Kosatsky, 2005; Fouillet et al, 2006). Around 60 per cent of these deaths were in people aged 75 and over (Confalonieri et al, 2007, p397). People living alone were also at higher risk of mortality (Fouillet et al, 2006). Other European countries, including Spain, Italy and the UK, were also affected (Kovats and Ebi, 2006). Extensive forest fires occurred in Portugal resulting in exposure of the affected population to harmful atmospheric pollution (NASA Visible Earth, 2003). Estimates suggest that there were around 2000 extra deaths in the UK (Johnson et al, 2005).

Deaths associated with heatwaves are not confined to the temperate zone. More than 3000 deaths were reported in Andhra Pradesh, India, in 2003 when the state experienced the most severe and longest heatwave in its recorded history with the temperature rising to 48.8°C (Rao, 2005). Heatwaves in South

Box 2.2
Key points: Heatwaves are occurring more frequently worldwide and are increasing the risks of:

- mortality in the elderly, the isolated, the young, outdoor workers and rural populations;
- increased deaths and injury due to forest fires.

Asia have been associated with high mortality in rural populations, the young, the elderly and outdoor workers (BBC News, 2002).

Extreme weather events

The IPCC estimates that some weather events and extremes will become more frequent, more widespread and/or more intense during this century (IPCC, 2007).

In the summer of 2007, England witnessed the wettest summer since records began, with extreme levels of rainfall compressed into relatively short periods of time. 55,000 properties were flooded, 7000 people had to be rescued from the flood waters by emergency services and 13 people died (Pitt Review, 2008, pIX). The loss of essential services was the largest since the Second World War with almost 0.5 million people left without mains water or electricity (Pitt Review, 2008, pIX). To put this event into context, there were over 200 major floods worldwide in 2007 affecting 800 million people and costing more than 8000 lives and over £40 billion damage.

Floods and tropical cyclones have the greatest impact in South Asia and Latin America and, in common with such extreme events elsewhere, result in deaths from drowning, unsafe or unhealthy conditions and injury. It is mainly low- and middle-income countries with poor sanitation and lack of safe water that report increased risks of diarrhoeal diseases, cholera, cryptosporidiosis and typhoid fever (Confalonieri et al, 2007, p398) in such circumstances. However, the diarrhoeal illness and deaths that resulted from water contamination following Hurricane Katrina are a fitting reminder that high-income countries are not immune from a breakdown of essential services in the aftermath of severe weather events (CDC, 2005).

Dangerous chemical contamination may result from flooding as was the case following Hurricane Katrina (Manuel, 2006), the worst natural disaster in the United States in 75 years, which killed more than 1000 people, uprooted 500,000 others and caused more than $100 billion worth of damage (Galea et al, 2007). Increasing population density in close proximity to industrial developments in many parts of the world greatly enhances the risk of mass human exposure to dangerous chemicals following an extreme weather event in the future.

Children living in rural poverty and urban slums with inadequate public water supply and sanitation facilities in the poorer parts of the world are most at risk of diarrhoeal disease and mortality, but very heavy rainfall may overwhelm water and sewage treatment and water drainage systems in any part of the world. Associations between extreme rainfall and outbreaks of water-borne diseases, and seasonal contamination of surface water and sporadic cases of diseases such as cryptosporidiosis and campylobacteriosis have been reported from North America and Europe (Curriero et al, 2001; Clark et al, 2003; Lake et al, 2005). One study of the health impact of floods in England in 2000 revealed a significant increase in self-reported risk of gastroenteritis (Reacher et al, 2004).

There is increasing recognition of two types of impacts that are common to all countries: the greater vulnerability and higher health burden of poorer communities that experience a weather disaster and the high levels of mental disorders (Confalonieri et al, 2007, p399). Exposure to hurricane-related stressors such as the death of a loved one, physical illness or injury and housing adversity was found to be widespread in a US study that explored the prevalence of mental illness in areas affected by Hurricane Katrina (Galea et al, 2007). The stressors played a critical role in the high prevalence of hurricane-related anxiety-mood disorders.

Coastal communities are particularly vulnerable to climate change because of the risk of storm surges, tropical cyclones and hurricanes exacerbated by the

Box 2.3
Key points: Extreme weather events

- Are becoming more frequent, more widespread and more intense.
- Are resulting in deaths, disease and injury due to drowning, lack of sanitation and safe drinking water and exposure to dangerous chemical contaminants.
- Are associated with high prevalence of mental illness.
- Result in enormous damage and economic loss.
- Impose a higher health burden on the poor.

accelerated rise in sea level (Confalonieri et al, 2007, p414). The challenges faced by such populations are described in greater detail later in the chapter.

Against a background of rising ambient temperatures, climate instability has the potential to precipitate ice and snow storms, making winter travel more hazardous (Epstein and Mills, 2005, p29) and increasing mortality even in countries adapted to the cold, because of disruptions in electricity or heating systems (Confalonieri et al, 2007, p398).

Air quality and disease

The weather is an important determinant of air quality. Some weather patterns may exacerbate the development of secondary chemical pollutants. Ground-level ozone occurs naturally and is also a constituent of urban smog. Its concentration has been increasing in most parts of the world. Because ozone formation depends on bright sunshine with high temperatures, concentrations are usually highest in the summer months. Exposure to high levels of ground-level ozone is associated with pneumonia, chronic obstructive pulmonary disease, asthma, allergic rhinitis and with premature mortality (Ebi and McGregor, 2008).

Weather patterns resulting from climate change are also associated with changing concentrations of other air pollutants such as fine particulate matter, which is known to increase morbidity and mortality (Confalonieri et al, 2007, p402). Changes in temperature and precipitation are increasing the frequency and severity of forest fires and the associated risks of burns, injuries and damage due to smoke inhalation. Air pollutants released by such events can be

Box 2.4
Key points: Air quality

- Climate change is an important determinant of air quality.
- Poor air quality is associated with higher levels of respiratory and cardiovascular disease.

transported great distances by changing wind patterns, and increase the risks of acute and chronic respiratory disease and mortality from respiratory as well as cardiovascular disease (Confalonieri et al, 2007, p402). Studies have also demonstrated increased mortality from cardiovascular and respiratory disease following a dust storm (Kwon et al, 2002).

Aeroallergens and disease

Climate change has resulted in the pollen season starting earlier in the northern hemisphere, extending the length of the season for some species only and increasing the concentration of other pollens (Confalonieri et al, 2007, p402). The incidence of pollen-induced allergenic diseases such as allergic rhinitis is showing changes reflective of these altered seasons. The self-reported prevalence of asthma increased 75 per cent from 1980 to 1994 in American adults and children (Rogers, 2005, p48). Large numbers of people also suffer from allergic rhinitis, making allergic diseases an important cause of chronic disease in the US (Rogers, 2005, p48). Allergic diseases have a strong genetic component, but the rapidity of the rise in prevalence is believed to point to air pollution and allergen exposure acting synergistically to increase the risk. New invasive plant species such as ragweed with highly allergenic pollen resulting in substantial health risks are spreading to several parts of the world, where

Box 2.5
Key points: Aeroallergens and disease

In the northern hemisphere:

- The pollen season is starting earlier and lasting longer.
- Pollen concentrations are higher and highly allergenic pollen from new plant species presents substantial health risks.
- Increased CO_2 and ambient temperatures are altering the timing, production and distribution of pollens.
- The prevalence of allergenic diseases such as asthma and rhinitis has increased in many countries.

increasing CO_2 concentrations and temperatures are conducive to greater production of pollen and a prolonged pollen season (Wayne et al, 2002).

Drought, nutrition and food security

Climate change is associated with both acute and chronic nutritional deficiency. Food and water shortage due to drought can directly result in death or severe under-nutrition. Under-nutrition itself can lead to greater vulnerability to infectious disease and greater risk of dying from it. Drought may trigger mass migrations as rural communities in particular search for safe water, food and livelihoods. Population displacements can lead to overcrowding and lack of safe water, food and shelter, further increasing the risk of malnutrition and vulnerability to communicable diseases and mental illness.

As the effects of climate change gradually increase, environmental refugees are likely to grow in numbers and may trigger resentment in host countries because of the pressures on their resources and this may precipitate climate wars in the future. There are 46 countries that are home to the world's poorest communities (Smith and Vivekananda, 2007) and at the greatest risk of violent conflict as a result of climate change reinforcing existing social, economic and political instability. The war and resulting human tragedy in Darfur, Sudan, is recognized as the first example, the conflict having been triggered by an ecological crisis resulting at least in part from climate change (Smith and Vivekananda, 2007).

In India, crop failures due to drought have driven farmers to suicide (Oxfam, 2008). Farmers in Australia too, are reported to be at higher risk of suicide during periods of drought (Nicholls et al, 2005).

The IPCC has also highlighted that 'the spatial distribution, intensity and seasonality of meningococcal meningitis appear to be strongly linked to climatic and environmental factors, particularly drought, although the causal mechanism is not clearly understood' (Confalonieri et al, 2007, p400). The report also states that in West Africa, the geographical distribution of meningitis has widened and this may be attributable in part to climate change. Drought is also associated with dust storms and consequent respiratory disease.

Water

An estimated 1.2 billion people worldwide, mainly in low- and middle-income countries, lack access to safe water (CSDH, 2008). Drought further reduces access to safe water and adds to the burden of diarrhoeal disease because of insufficient and contaminated water. Persistent diarrhoea and consequent chronic malnutrition in children are important risk factors for high levels of childhood mortality in many parts of the world, such as sub-Saharan Africa (Confalonieri et al, 2007, p401).

Changes in water quality due to low river flows are not confined to the developing world, as confirmed by observations from The Netherlands during a dry summer in 2003 (Senhorst and Zwolsman, 2005). A UK Government report in 2008 highlights that there is relatively little water available per person in parts of England, particularly in the south-east and in urban areas. Contrary to Britain's popular image of a wet and green land, its population density is high and existing abstraction is causing unacceptable damage to the environment (DEFRA, 2008).

Food security

Global food prices have risen sharply in recent years (BBC News, 2008). Higher food prices are likely to undermine the diet of the poor both in terms of quantity and nutritional quality. The developed countries have not been immune to this, as was demonstrated by the rise in food prices in the UK in 2007 (Higham, 2007). But the most serious consequences are inevitably being felt in the poorest regions of the developing world. Health and social inequalities are likely to increase as a result, both within and between countries. In some parts of the world, increasing food prices have resulted in political unrest. Food riots such as in Haiti where food prices increased by 50–100 per cent are projected to become more common (BBC News, 2008).

The immediate factors thought to have influenced this escalation in food prices include droughts in major wheat-producing countries in recent years, as well as diversion of 5 per cent of the world's cereals to biofuels. Both issues have a link with climate change. More volatile weather patterns are projected as a result of climate change and are expected to increase in their negative impact on agricultural production worldwide (Von Braun, 2008). Furthermore, the search

Box 2.6
Key points: Drought associated with climate change:

- May result in food and water shortage, which could lead to:

  - severe under-nutrition and greater vulnerability to infectious disease;
  - population displacements and mass migrations with all the associated health risks;
  - environmental refugees and climate conflict.

- May lead to crop failures driving farmers to suicide.
- May be linked to changes in the distribution, intensity and seasonality of meningococcal meningitis.
- May add to the burden of diarrhoeal disease in countries already lacking access to safe water.
- May increase global food prices.

driven by the developed world for plant-derived fuels to reduce dependence on fossil fuels and the resulting greenhouse gas emissions is increasing the risks of food crises worldwide.

Food safety

There is a clear correlation between rising temperatures and the incidence of common forms of food poisoning such as salmonellosis (Kovats et al, 2004). Even in the UK, additional food poisoning notifications of 4000, 9000 and 14,000 are projected for +1°C, +2°C and +3°C increases in temperature (DH/HPA, 2008, p74). Warmer weather also increases the numbers of flies, rodents and other pests that have the potential to contaminate food. Warming of the seas is increasing the risk of shellfish poisoning, mainly due to contamination by toxin-producing algal blooms (Hallegraeff, 2008).

Although occurring naturally, mercury is a global pollutant and a serious public health concern when elevated above natural background levels. Mercury in rivers, lakes and oceans converts into the most poisonous form, methylmercury, and builds up in fish, with predatory fish at the top of the food chain being most contaminated. Methylation rates are temperature dependent and are increasing due to climate change (Booth and Zeller, 2005). A United Nations Environment Programme Report published in 2003 (UNEP, 2003) has highlighted the increasing health risks being faced by people worldwide who eat fish, but especially those populations particularly dependent on marine resources for food, such as the inhabitants of the Faroe Islands and the Arctic region.

Climate change and the consequent increase in water temperatures and salinity observed in aquatic environments close to the Bay of Bengal are creating more favourable conditions for the multiplication of aquatic reservoirs of cholera. Combined with poor sanitation, this is not only resulting in the risk of cholera in remote coastal villages in the mangrove area of Bangladesh, but is also increasing the risk of an epidemic spread of cholera (ICDDR, B, 2007).

In India, drought conditions in the summer often result in power crises in many states dependent on hydroelectric power, rendering refrigeration systems non-functional and increasing the risk of food poisoning (Healthy-India.org).

Box 2.7
Key points: How climate change may compromise food safety

- Warmer temperatures increase the incidence of food poisoning.
- Warming of the seas may stimulate toxin-producing algal blooms that can contaminate shellfish.
- Mercury levels may build up in fish and increase the health risks of consumers.
- Rising temperatures are increasing the risk of cholera in Bangladesh and enhancing the risk of epidemic spread.

Vector-borne, rodent-borne and other infectious diseases

Major shifts in patterns and distribution of vector-borne diseases are anticipated in association with climate change. Tick-borne encephalitis is an
important vector-borne disease in Europe. Based on changes that are already
occurring, studies of the tick-borne encephalitis virus suggest that its distribution may expand both north and west of Stockholm, Sweden, but conversely
its inherent fragility may put its survival at risk in other areas as the climate
becomes warmer (Randolph and Rogers, 2000). In Canada, due to climate
warming, ticks are expected to spread northward into areas that were previously tick free (CCDR, 2008).

Lyme disease is the most prevalent vector-borne disease in the USA and has
spread throughout the north-east and parts of the north-central and north-
west of the country since it was discovered in 1977 (Brownstein, 2005, p45).
It is caused by the bacteria *Borrelia burgdorferi* and the vector is the deer tick.
Whilst treatable with antibiotics, untreated infection can affect the nervous
and musculoskeletal systems and the heart and can cause chronic disability.
Although factors such as reforestation are the most likely explanations for the
increased prevalence of Lyme disease, climate is likely to also play a part.

Malaria kills more than a million people worldwide each year – 90 per cent
of them in Africa (Molavi, 2003). Modelling based on current associations
between the occurrence of disease and climatic conditions has been used to
show that small temperature and humidity increases can greatly affect the
potential for malaria transmission. Areas previously at little risk may become
malaria prone, while others that currently experience outbreaks may see
a reduction in transmission. Warming increases the rate of reproduction of
mosquitoes, boosts biting and prolongs their breeding season (Epstein, 2005).
Globally, temperature increases of 2–3°C may increase the number of people
who, in climatic terms, are at risk of malaria by around 3 to 5 per cent, that is,
several hundred million (WHO, 2003). Floods and heavy rainfall may increase
the risk of malaria by expanding mosquito breeding sites and droughts by triggering population migrations into and out of areas with malaria.

Some countries that currently do not experience malaria may see increased
occurrences as conditions become more favourable for transmission. Climate

change scenarios suggest an increase in the theoretical risk of malaria transmission in the south of England where the salt marshes are home to some types of mosquitoes, as well as spreading north to the Scottish borders, if the climate becomes warmer (DH/HPA, 2008, p42).

Dengue is also one of the world's most important vector-borne diseases with about 30 per cent of the world's population living in areas where the climate is suitable for its transmission (Hales et al, 2002). It is caused by a virus transmitted by the bite of infected *Aedes aegypti* mosquitoes. Symptoms of dengue fever usually subside within a few days, but dengue haemorrhagic fever, which has a much higher fatality rate especially in children and immune suppressed individuals, may develop in a few cases. By 2085, it is projected that 50 to 60 per cent of the global population would be at risk because of climate change (Hales et al, 2002) and that the significantly increased population at risk would include countries such as Australia (McMichael et al, 2006) and New Zealand (De Wet et al, 2001).

The risk of infectious diseases transmitted by rodents may increase during heavy rains and flooding (WHO, 2005b). In Brazil, living near an open sewer or workplace where there is exposure to flood or sewer water has been demonstrated to be a risk factor for developing leptospirosis in urban populations (Sarkar et al, 2002). This infectious bacterial disease can vary in presentation from mild to severe, and potentially fatal, illness. It is transmitted by contact with urine from infected animals, as well as through water contaminated by, for example, urine from rats and mice.

Climate instability is also contributing to the emergence of infectious diseases along bird migratory pathways. West Nile Virus (WNV) infection is an important example of such a disease, which can affect birds, animals and humans (Epstein and Causey, 2005). The *Culex pipiens* mosquito is the primary vector for WNV and thrives in stagnant pools of water particularly in urban areas. These mosquitoes bite birds and infect them. Droughts combined with warm temperatures increase viral development both in the mosquitoes and in birds. Shrinking water sites in periods of drought also concentrate the numbers of birds increasingly seen in urban areas, as well as the bird-biting mosquitoes, further increasing the chance of mosquito–bird viral transmission. Thus the stage is set in drought affected urban areas for humans to become infected.

WNV disease first appeared in the USA in 1999 when an outbreak in New York City resulted in 62 people developing encephalitis (inflammation of the brain) and meningoenchephalitis (inflammation of the brain and its covering), of whom 7 died (Epstein and Causey, 2005, p42). Warm temperatures accompanying droughts are thought to be responsible for outbreaks in subsequent years that have affected thousands of people. Outbreaks have also occurred in many other countries in Europe and Africa. More frequent droughts and warmer temperatures in the future may increase WNV infection rates (Epstein and Causey, 2005, p44).

Box 2.8
Key points: Major shifts in patterns and distribution of vector-borne diseases are anticipated in association with climate change

- Some northward expansion of tick-borne disease is projected in parts of Europe, Canada and the US but, conversely, warming may put the survival of ticks at risk in other areas.
- Globally, temperature increases of 2–3°C may increase the number of people who in climatic terms are at risk of malaria by around 3 to 5 per cent, that is, several hundred million.
- By 2085, it is projected that 50 to 60 per cent of the global population would be at risk of dengue because of climate change.
- Prolonged drought and resulting crop failures are resulting in rural–urban migration of people and increasing the risk of transmission of vector-borne diseases.
- Heavy rains and flooding are increasing the risk of diseases such as leptospirosis transmitted by rodents.
- Climate instability is also contributing to the emergence of infectious diseases such as West Nile Virus disease along bird migratory pathways.

Ultraviolet radiation and health

'Scientists 100 years ago would have been incredulous at the idea that, by the late twentieth century, humankind would be affecting the stratosphere. Yet, remarkably, human-induced depletion of stratospheric ozone has recently begun – after 8,000 generations of Homo sapiens' (WHO, 2003).

Strictly speaking, stratospheric ozone depletion is not part of 'global climate change' that occurs in the troposphere. There are, however, several recently described interactions between ozone depletion and greenhouse gas induced warming (WHO, 2003).

'Ozone affects climate and climate affects ozone' (Allen, 2004). Stratospheric ozone (which is different from ground-level ozone) absorbs much of the incoming solar ultraviolet radiation (UVR), especially the biologically more damaging, shorter-wavelength, UVR. Industrial halogenated chemicals such as the chlorofluorocarbons (CFCs – used in refrigeration, insulation and spray-can propellants), while inert at ambient Earth-surface temperatures, destroy the ozone in the extremely cold polar stratosphere, especially in late winter and early spring (WHO, 2003). In 1987, recognition of the dangers of ozone deple-tion led to the adoption worldwide of the Montreal Protocol, intended to stop the use of such chemicals. As a consequence, recovery of the stratospheric ozone was anticipated by the middle of the 21st century (WHO, 2003), but the effects of climate change may prolong this (Confalonieri et al, 2007, p405). Rising atmospheric temperatures are resulting in chemical processes that deplete stratospheric ozone and, as a result, exposures to UVR are anticipated to peak in parts of the world such as Europe by 2020.

Box 2.9
Key points: Ultraviolet radiation (UVR) and health

- Warming is resulting in chemical processes which deplete stratospheric ozone and, as a result, exposure to UVR.
- Adverse effects of excess exposure to UVR include skin cancers, sunburn, cataracts and a weakened immune response to immunizations.

UVR exposure is essential for the production of vitamin D in the body, but excess exposure has mainly adverse impacts on health. According to IPCC estimates, UVR exposure caused 60,000 premature deaths in 2000 (Prüss-Üstun et al, 2006). The most important health effects are cutaneous malignant melanoma, non-melanocytic skin cancers, sunburn, UVR induced cataracts and weakened immune responses to immunizations (Prüss-Üstun et al, 2006). White populations are most vulnerable to skin cancer and contemporary life-styles and choices in relation to clothes and prolonged sun exposure enhance the risk (WHO, 2003).

Occupational health

Climate change poses substantial threats to occupational health and safety (Confalonieri et al, 2007, p405). Workers, irrespective of whether they work outdoors or indoors, may be at risk of severe heat-related illness and even death because of rising temperatures and humidity. Heatwaves put workers at particular risk and this risk is spread across the world, as studies from the US as well as South Asia have shown. (Krake et al, 2003; OCHA, 2003). The mental health impacts of climate change-related agricultural disasters on the farming community are well documented (Nicholls et al, 2005; Oxfam, 2008).

Box 2.10
Key points: Climate change poses substantial threats to occupational health and safety

- Indoor and outdoor workers are at risk of heat-related illness associated with heatwaves.
- Agricultural disasters are associated with adverse mental health impacts in the farming community.
- Emergency and rescue workers are at increasing risk of injury and deaths, due to more frequent, more widespread and more intense weather events.

Populations at particular risk

People living in coastal areas

An Oxfam report published in 2008 confirmed that the island of Lohachara in the Sunderbans delta along the Bay of Bengal previously inhabited by 10,000 people was the first island to be submerged by rising sea levels in 2006 (Oxfam, 2008, p13), a fact unlikely to be known to many in the parts of the world with the highest levels of greenhouse gas emissions. A vulnerability assessment of the Sunderbans island system in the context of climate change projected that a dozen islands, inhabited by about 70,000 people, are at risk of disappearing by 2030 (Greenpeace, 2007).

About 60 per cent of the world population lives within 100 kilometres of the coastline (UNEP, 1997). The recognized effects of climate change impacting on the health of coastal populations include coastal flooding, increasing contamination due to rising sea temperatures, increasing salinity of coastal fresh waters, and dramatically declining fish populations (Confalonieri et al, 2007, p414). Small Island States are particularly vulnerable (WHO, 2005a). By the turn of the century the Maldives, with 80 per cent of its islands lying less than one metre above sea level, will be uninhabitable, forcing most of its population to be displaced (Oxfam, 2008).

Other low-lying areas, particularly in the densely populated region of South Asia, are also heavily at risk. A rise of more than 2°C is expected to further increase coastal flooding in Bangladesh, with the added risk that salt water will infiltrate drinking water (Oxfam, 2008).

Populations in polar regions

The health of the indigenous populations living in the polar regions is already substantially affected by climate change. Rising winter temperatures are projected to reduce excess winter deaths from cardiovascular and respiratory disease (Confalonieri et al, 2007, p415). However, rising temperatures are also projected to lengthen the season for disease transmission by wildlife and insects in some areas (Bradley et al, 2005). In Alaska, walking on thinning ice is resulting in an increase in accidents among Inuits (Epstein, 2005).

Food security has some unique features in relation to the Aboriginal communities in Canada, with 'cultural' food security being an additional dimension (Power, 2008). This notion relates to the harvesting, sharing and consumption of traditional foods, primarily wild-harvested foods such as wild meat, fish, birds, sea mammals and berries and other plants. The impact of climate change on natural systems and the resulting environmental contamination is affecting the availability, supply and safety of traditional foods. Market foods, which are less nutritious, are therefore replacing traditional foods in the diet of such communities, with effects on both physical and mental health, and indeed, survival itself (Power, 2008).

Populations living in mountain regions

Mountain glaciers are in retreat with ice and snow melting at an alarming rate in all mountainous regions of the world. The Gangotri glacier in the Himalayas is the source of water for the river Ganges. With climate change, the glacier is retreating at the speed of about 30 metres a year. With continued warming it will melt rapidly, initially releasing large volumes of water. But in the long term there may be little water left (Government of India, 2001). Communities that are dependent on seasonal melting of ice for fresh water could face water insecurity in the long term, with the projected declines in glacial melt in places such as India (Government of India, 2001) and China (Confalonieri et al, 2007, p414).

Conclusion

In the year 2000, climate change was estimated to have caused over 150,000 deaths worldwide (WHO, 2005a). Even if an early and rapid decline in green-house gas emissions is achieved, temperatures are likely to continue to rise, because carbon dioxide in the atmosphere will remain for many years to come and the climate takes some time to respond to changes (Pope, 2008). With natural systems continuing to be affected on a daily basis, major risks to health will remain for the foreseeable future.

Climate change is already exerting serious adverse effects on the health of communities in both developing and developed countries. Improving popula-tion health and well-being may be the most persuasive basis for collective action to address the risks we face worldwide from continuing climate change, as we shall propose in detail in Chapter 4.

References

Allen, J. (2004) 'Tango in the Atmosphere: Ozone and Climate Change', available at http://earthobservatory.nasa.gov/Features/Tango/ (accessed 28 January 2009)

BBC News (2002) 'Heat 'kills 450' in Southern India', *BBC News Online*, available at http://news.bbc.co.uk/2/hi/south_asia/1991215.stm (accessed 11 February 2009)

BBC News (2008) 'World Bank tackles food emergency', *BBC News Online*, available at http://news.bbc.co.uk/go/pr/fr/-/2/hi/business/7344892.stm, 2008 (accessed 12 February 2009)

Bhattacharya, S. (2003) 'European heatwave caused 35,000 deaths', *New Scientist*, available at www.newscientist.com/article/dn4259-european-heatwave-caused-35000-deaths.html (accessed 28 January 2009)

Booth, S. and Zeller, D. (2005) 'Mercury, food webs, and marine mammals: implications of diet and climate change for human health', *Environmental Health Perspectives*, available at www.ehponline.org/members/2005/7603/7603.pdf (accessed 11 February 2009)

Bradley M.J., Kutz, S.J, Jenkins E. and O'Hara, T.M. (2005) 'The potential impact of climate change on infectious disease of arctic fauna', *Int. J. Circumpolar Health*, vol 64, pp468–477

Brownstein, J. (2005) Lyme Disease: Implications of climate change', in Epstein, P.R. and Mills, E. (eds) *Climate Change Futures, Health, Ecological and Economic Dimensions,* The Center for Health and the Global Environment, Harvard Medical School, pp45–47

CCDR (2008) 'The rising challenge of Lyme borreliosis in Canada', vol 34, no 1, available at www.phac-aspc.gc.ca/publicat/ccdr-rmtc/08vol34/dr-rm3401a-eng.php (accessed 11 February 2009)

CDC (2005) 'Vibrio illnesses after Hurricane Katrina: multiple states, August–September 2005', *MMWR–Morb.Mortal. Weekly Report*, vol 54, pp928–931

Clark, C.G., Price, L., Ahmed, R., Woodward, D.L., Melito, P.L., Rogers F.G., Jamieson, D., Ciebin, B., Li, A. and Ellis A. (2003) 'Characterization of water borne disease outbreak associated Campylobacter jejuni, Walkerton, Ontario', *Emerging Infectious Diseases*, vol 9, pp1232–1241

Confalonieri, U., Menne, B., Akhtar, R., Ebi, K.L., Hauengue, M., Kovats, R.S., Revich, B. and Woodward, A. (2007) 'Human Health: Climate Change 2007: Impacts, Adaptation and Vulnerability, Contribution of Working Group II to the Fourth Assessment Report of the Intergovernmental Panel on Climate Change', in

Parry, M. L., Canziani, O. F., Palutikof, J. P., van der Linden, P. J. and Hanson, C. E. (eds) Cambridge University Press, Cambridge, UK, pp391–431

CSDH (2008) 'Closing the Gap in a Generation: Health Equity Through Action on the Social Determinants of Health', Final Report of the Commission on Social Determinants of Health, World Health Organization, Geneva

Curriero, F., Patz, J.A., Rose, J.B., and Lele, S. (2001) 'The association between extreme precipitation and waterborne disease outbreaks in the United States, 1948–1994', American Journal of Public Health, vol 91, pp1194–1199

DEFRA (2008) 'Sustainable development indicators in your pocket 2008', an update of the UK Government Strategy indicators, Defra Publications, London, pp41–43

De Wet, N., Woodward, A. and Weinstein, P. (2001) 'Use of a computer model to identify potential hotspots for dengue fever in New Zealand', New Zealand Medical Journal., vol 114, pp420–422, available at http://cat.inist.fr/?aModele=afficheN&c psidt=14091296 (accessed 3 December 2008)

DH/HPA (2008) 'Health Effects of Climate Change in the UK', an update of the Department of Health report 2001/2002, Sari Kovats (ed)

Ebi, K.L. and McGregor, G. (2008) 'Climate change, tropospheric ozone and particulate health impacts', Environmental Health Perspectives, vol 116, no 11, pp1449–1455

Epstein, P.R. (2005) 'Climate change and human health', New England Journal of Medicine, vol 353, no 14, pp1433–1434

Epstein, P. and Causey, D. (2005) 'West Nile Virus: A disease of wildlife and a force of global change', in Epstein, P.R. and Mills, E. (eds) Climate Change Futures, Health, Ecological and Economic Dimensions, The Center for Health and the Global Environment, Harvard Medical School, pp41–44

Epstein, P.R. and Mills, E. (2005) Climate Change Futures, Health, Ecological and Economic Dimensions, The Center for Health and the Global Environment, Harvard Medical School

Fouillet, A., Rey, G., Laurent, F., Pavillon, G., Bellec, S., Guihenneuc-Jouyaux, C., Clavel, J., Jougla, E. and Hemon, D. (2006) 'Excess mortality related to the August 2003 heat wave in France', International Archives of Occupational and Environmental Health, vol 80, no 1, pp16–24

Galea, S., Brewin, C.R., Gruber, M., Jones, R.T., King, D.W., King, L.A., McNally, R.J., Ursano, R.J., Petukhova, M. and Kessler, R.C. (2007) 'Exposure to hurricane-related stressors and mental illness after Hurricane Katrina', Archives of General Psychiatry, vol 64, no 12, pp1427–1434

Government of India, Ministry of Environment & Forests (2001) 'Climate Change, Did you Know?', available at http://envfor.nic.in/cc/diduknow.htm (accessed 16 February 2009)

Greenpeace (2007) 'People of the Sunderbans take action to arrest sea level rise', available at www.greenpeace.org/india/press/releases/people-of-the-sunderban-s-take (accessed 13 February 2009)

Haines, A., Kovats, R.S., Lendrum-Campbell, D. and Corvalan, C. (2006) 'Climate change and human health: impacts, vulnerability, and mitigation', *The Lancet*, vol 367, pp2101–2109

Hales, S., De Wet, N., Maindonald, J. and Woodward, A. (2002) 'Potential effect of population and climate changes on global distribution of dengue fever: an empirical model', *The Lancet*, available at http://image.thelancet.com/extras/01art11175web.pdf (accessed 11 February 2009)

Hallegraeff, G. (2008) 'Impacts of climate change on harmful algal blooms, SciTopics, Research summaries by experts', available at http://scitopics.com/Impacts_of_Climate_Change_on_Harmful_Algal_Blooms.html (accessed 28 January 2009)

Healthy-India.org, Health through Hygiene, Eat Freshly Cooked Food, available at http://healthy-india.org/hygiene6.asp (accessed 11 February 2009)

Higham, N. (2007) 'Food prices on the rise and rise', *BBC NEWS*, available at http://news.bbc.co.uk/1/hi/uk/6909469.stm (accessed 28 January 2009)

HM Government (2008) *Health is global, a UK Government Strategy 2008–13 Annexes*, London

ICDDR, B (2007) International Centre for Diarrhoeal Disease Research, Bangladesh, available at www.icddrb.org/pub/publication.jsp?classificationID=46&pubID=9371 (accessed 11 February 2009)

IPCC (2001) 'IPCC Special Report on The Regional Impacts of Climate Change An Assessment of Vulnerability', Watson, R.T., Zinyowera, M.C., Moss, R.T., available at www.grida.no/publications/other/ipcc_sr/ (accessed 9 February 2009)

IPCC (2007) 'Summary for Policymakers', in Parry, M.L., Canziani, O.F., Palutikof, J.P., van der Linden, P.J. and Hanson, C.E. (eds) 'Climate Change 2007: Impacts, Adaptation and Vulnerability. Contribution of Working Group II to the Fourth Assessment Report of the Intergovernmental Panel on Climate Change', Cambridge University, Cambridge, UK, pp7–22

Johnson, H., Kovats, R.S., McGregor, G., Stedman, J., Gibbs, M., Walton, H., Cook, I. and Black, E. (2005) 'The impact of the 2003 heat wave on mortality and hospital admissions in England', *National Statistics, Health Statistics Quarterly*, no 25, pp6–11

Kosatsky, T. (2005) 'The 2003 European Heat Waves', *Eurosurveillance*, vol 10, no 7, p552, available at www.eurosurveillance.org/ViewArticle.aspx?ArticleId=552 (accessed 28 January 2009)

Kovats, R.S., Hajat, S., Edwards, S., Armstrong, B., Ebi, K.L. and Menne, B. (Collaborating Group) (2004) 'The effect of temperature on food poisoning: a time series analysis of salmonellosis in 10 European populations', *Epidemiology and Infection*, vol 132, no 3, pp443–453

Kovats, R.S. and Ebi, K.L. (2006) 'Heatwaves and public health in Europe', *European Journal of Public Health*, vol 16, pp592–599; doi:10.1093/eurpub/ck1049

Krake, A., McCullough, J. and King, B. (2003) 'Health hazards to park rangers from excessive heat at Grand Canyon National Park', *Applied Occupational and Environmental Hygiene*, vol 18, pp295–317

Kwon, H.J., Cho, S.H., Chun, H., Lagarde, F. and Pershagen, G. (2002) 'Effects of Asian dust events on daily mortality in Seoul, Korea', *Environmental Research*, vol 90, pp1–5

Lake, I., Bentham, G., Kovats R.S. and Nichols, G. (2005) 'Effects of weather and the river flow on cryptosporidiosis', *Water Health*, vol 3, pp469–474

Lean, G. (2006) 'Disappearing world: Global warming claims tropical island', *The Independent*, available at www.independent.co.uk/environment/climate-change/disappearing-world-global-warming-claims-tropical-island-429764.html (accessed 28 January 2009)

Manuel, J. (2006) 'In Katrina's wake', *Environmental Health Perspectives*, vol 114, A32–A39

McMichael, A.J., Woodruff, R.E. and Hales, S. (2006) 'Climate change and human health: present and future risks', *The Lancet*, vol 367, pp859–869

McMichael, A.J., Friel, S., Nyong, A. and Corvalan, C. (2008) 'Global environmental change and health: impacts, inequalities, and the health sector', *British Medical Journal*, vol 336, pp191–194

Molavi, A. (2003) 'Africa's Malaria Death Toll Still "Outrageously High"', National Geographic News, available at http://news.nationalgeographic.com/news/2003/06/0612_030612_malaria.html (accessed 20 February 2009)

NASA Visible Earth (2003) 'Forest Fires In Portugal' (updated 8 June 2006), available at http://visibleearth.nasa.gov/view_rec.php?id=18772 (accessed 28 January 2009)

Nicholls, N., Butler, C. and Hanigan, I. (2005) 'Inter-annual rainfall variations and suicide in New South Wales, Australia, 1964 to 2001', *International Journal of Biometeorology*, vol 50, pp139–143

OCHA (2003) 'India: Heat Wave – Occurred: 20 May 2003–5 June 2003', OCHA Situation Report no. 1, available at http://iys.cidi.org/disaster/03a/ixl131.html (accessed 17 February 2009)

Oxfam International (2008) *Rethinking Disasters; why death and destruction is not nature's fault but human failure*, South Asia Regional Centre, Oxfam (India) Trust, New Delhi

Pitt Review (2008) 'Learning Lessons from the 2007 Floods', UK Government, available at http://archive.cabinetoffice.gov.uk/pittreview/thepittreview/final_report.html (accessed 11 February 2009)

Pope, V. (2008) 'Met Office's bleak forecast on climate change, The head of the Met Office centre for climate change research explains why the momentum on emissions targets must not be lost', *The Guardian*, available at www.guardian.co.uk/environment/2008/oct/01/climatechange.carbonemissions (accessed 11 February 2009)

Power Elaine, M. (2008) 'Conceptualizing food security for Aboriginal People in Canada', *Canadian Journal of Public Health*, vol 99, no 2, pp95–97

Prüss-Üstun, A., Zeeb, H., Mathers, C. and Repacholi, M. (eds) (2006) *Solar Ultraviolet Radiation: Global Burden of Disease from Ultraviolet Radiation*. Environmental Burden of Disease Series, vol 13, World Health Organization, Geneva, p285

Randolph, S.E. and Rogers, D.J. (2000) 'Fragile transmission cycles of tick-borne encephalitis virus may be disrupted by predicted climate change', *Proceedings of the Royal Society B: Biological Sciences*, vol 267, pp1741–1744

Rao, M. M. (2005) 'No early let-up in heat wave', *The Hindu*, available at: www.hindu.com/2005/05/22/stories/2005052210190400.htm (accessed 28 January 2009)

Reacher, M., McKenzie K., Lane C., Nichols T., Kedge I., Iverson A., Hepple P., Walter T., Laxton C. and Simpson J. (on behalf of the Lewes Flood Action Recovery Team) (2004) 'Health Impacts of Flooding in Lewes: a comparison of reported gastrointestinal and other illness and mental health in flooded and non-flooded households', *Communicable Disease and Public Health*, vol 7, no 1, pp 1–8, available at www.hpa.org.uk/web/HPAwebFile/HPAwebC/1213773807525 (accessed 11 February 2009)

Rogers, C.A. (2005) 'Carbon dioxide and aeroallergens', in Epstein, P.R. and Mills, E. (eds) *Climate Change Futures, Health, Ecological and Economic Dimensions*, The Center for Health and the Global Environment, Harvard Medical School, pp48–52

Sarkar, U., Nascimento, S.F., Barbosa, R., Martins, R., Nuevo, H., Kalafanos, I., Grunstein, I., Flannery, B., Dias, J., Riley, L.W., Reis, M.G. and Ko., A.I. (2002) 'Population-based case-control investigation of risk factors for leptospirosis during an urban epidemic', *American Journal of Tropical Medicine and Hygiene*, vol 66, no 5, pp605–610

Senhorst, H.A. and Zwolsman, J.J. (2005) 'Climate change and effects on water quality: a first impression', *Water Science and Technology*, vol 51, pp53–59

Smith, D. and Vivekananda, J. (2007) 'A climate of conflict: the links between climate change, peace and war', *International Alert*, London

Spratt, D. and Sutton, P. (2008) '3 Degrees of Warming', extract from 'Climate "Code Red" The Case for a Sustainability Emergency', available at www.global-greenhouse-warming.com/3-degrees.html (accessed 28 January 2009)

UNDP (2005) 'International Cooperation at a Crossroads: Aid, Trade and Security in an Unequal World', Human Development Report 2005, UNDP

UNECA (2006) 'Report on Climate Change, 2006', African Regional Implementation Review for the 14th Session of the Commission on Sustainable Development (CSD-14), prepared by UNEP, available at www.uneca.org/csd/CSD4_Report_on_Climate_Change.htm (accessed on 9 February 2009)

UNEP (1997) 'Global Environment Outlook – 1: Executive Summary: Overview of Regional Status and Trends', available at www.unep.org/geo/geo1/exsum/ex3.htm (accessed 17 February 2009)

UNEP (2003) 'Power Stations Threaten People and Wildlife with Mercury Poisoning', UNEP News Release, available at www.unep.org/Documents.Multilingual/Default.asp?DocumentID=284&ArticleID=3204&l=en (accessed 11 February 2009)

Von Braun, J. (2008) 'High and Rising Food Prices', in USAID conference, 'Addressing the Challenges of a Changing World Food Situation: Preventing Crisis and Leveraging Opportunity', Washington, DC, 11 April 2008

Wayne, P., Foster, S., Connolly, J., Bazzaz, F. and Epstein, P. (2002) 'Production of allergenic pollen by ragweed (*Ambrosia artemisiifolia* L.) is increased in CO_2-enriched atmospheres', *Annals of Allergy, Asthma and Immunology*, vol 88, no 3, pp279–282

WHO (2003) 'Climate change and human health – risks and responses', Summary, ISBN 9241590815, available at www.who.int/globalchange/climate/summary/en/index6.html (accessed 11 February 2009)

WHO (2005a) 'Climate and health, Fact Sheet', July 2005, available at www.who.int/globalchange/news/fsclimandhealth/en/print.html (accessed 11 February 2009)

WHO (2005b) 'Flooding and communicable diseases Fact Sheet, risk assessment and preventive measures', available at www.helid.desastres.net/?e=d-010who--000--1-0--010---4-----0--0-10l--11en-5000---50-about-0---01131-001-110utfZz-8-0-0&a=d&c=who&cl=CL4&d=Js8231e.1 (accessed 28 January 2009)

3 Health and the Natural Environment

David Stone

Humankind has not woven the web of life. We are but one thread within it. Whatever we do to the web, we do to ourselves. All things are bound together. All things connect.

Chief Seattle, 1855

Summary

A wide range of factors with complex interactions influence human health. The evidence is strong that contact with and access to natural environments are good for people's physical and mental health. More widely, the natural environment and global ecosystems have a huge influence on health, through 'ecosystem services' that are utilized by humans. These services include products like food and fuel, breathable air and supplies of potable water. The most recent United Nations Environment Programme Global Environment Outlook reports substantial change to the global and local environments that determine our health. There is a general deterioration in air quality, unsustainable use of land and water resources and substantial declines in biodiversity. The functionality of ecosystem processes is stressed almost to breaking point, due to pressure by people. Climate change will increase the rate of environmental change, exacerbating this situation. The consequences of the destruction and degradation of the environment for individual and population health are already with us in high levels of mortality due to environmental causes, such as air pollution. Sustainable development is the aspiration that the drive for social justice, health equality, environmental justice and economic development within the limits of available natural resources, can all come together.

Key terms

Anthropocentric: A perspective that views humanity as the centre of the universe.

Anthropogenic: Pertaining to the effect of human beings on the natural world.

Ecology: Study of the interactions between plants, animals, peoples and their environment.

Ecosystem: An ecosystem is a dynamic complex of plant, animal, and micro-organism communities and the nonliving environment, interacting as a functional unit. People are an integral part of ecosystems (MEA, 2003).

Ecosystem services: The benefits people obtain from ecosystems which include environmental resources and produce (MEA, 2003).

Introduction

As we have seen in Chapter 1, there is unequivocal evidence that climate change is taking place. It is being driven largely by emissions that are anthropogenic in origin. Critically, climatic change is altering the global ecosystem at an unprecedented rate and this may have profound effects on human health unless we can prevent it from getting worse. In this chapter we shall explore the relationship between the natural environment and human health and the possible consequences of altering that relationship as the impact of climate change worsens.

Health and its determinants

What determines our health? In fact, what do we mean by the term health? A quick look at a dictionary exposes terms like 'wholesomeness', 'soundness', and 'bodily condition'. Most health practitioners will ponder these fundamental questions from time to time and there can be little doubt that the answers are not straightforward. However, a brief consideration here will help shed light on why natural environments are important to our well-being.

The biological systems and processes of the human body are complex. Our bodies respond in many different ways to the positive and negative stimuli they experience, such as energy inputs (i.e. food), and biological invasions (e.g. viruses). Our understanding of health goes beyond the functioning of our biological systems and processes: a sound bodily condition. The classical definition of health was conceived as part of the founding constitution of the World Health Organization (WHO). WHO defines health as 'a state of complete physical, mental and social well-being and not merely the absence of disease or infirmity' (WHO, 2005a). Whilst there are some ambiguities and problems within this definition, it is long-standing and widely accepted, and importantly it embodies the idea that external environments as well as biological responses determine the health of a person.

Accepting this broad definition of health, we then need to consider what influences individual and community health outcomes. What determines our health? During the 1990s differences in health outcomes became of increasing concern to public health practitioners and academics alike. Despite decades of investment and advances in medical science, differences or inequalities in health outcomes existed across society. Dahlgren and Whitehead (1991) explored the underlying reasons for these inequalities and in doing so developed a model of health determinants that has become a foundation of public health in developed countries. Their model made the assertion that the expected health outcomes for an individual were influenced by more than just genetics. They reasoned that a range of influences – lifestyle, social, cultural and economic – determine individual and community health and that the differences in these factors drive inequalities in health.

An example of the determinants of health: Obesity

The increasing prevalence of obesity amongst the adult population is a serious public health concern in many countries. In 2006, 24 per cent of adults in England were classified as obese (The Information Centre, 2008). Obesity is often cited as resulting from lifestyle, that is to say individual choices about diet and physical activity. The causes of obesity are not quite so simple though. Other factors or determinants influence the individual and their lifestyle choices. An unemployed person, let us call him Mr Jay, living in a deprived neighbourhood with few fresh food outlets, will have limited access to healthy choices with respect to diet and activity. This simplified example illustrates the complex interplay between the factors that determine health.

Dahlgren and Whitehead's model extended only as far as individual life and working condition determinants: factors that might be considered manipulable by changes in social or economic policy, which was their particular interest. Growing knowledge about the determinants of health, learning from the WHO Healthy Cities initiative (see Chapter 6), and consideration of the ambitious goals set by the United Nations World Summit on Sustainable Development (Johannesburg, 2002) prompted Barton and Grant (2006) to extend the classical determinants model incorporating built and natural, local and global, environmental determinants of health.

Going back to our simplified obesity example of Mr Jay, unemployed and living in a neighbourhood without grocers, what difference might consideration of environmental determinants make to the underlying reasons for his obesity? We may find the neighbourhood has heavy traffic, few footpaths and cycle paths, poor public transport and lacks public open spaces, all of which act as barriers to increasing physical activity. These determinants are less direct, but no less important, in influencing the health of Mr Jay. If he cannot easily be physically active or move about within his neighbourhood, he has multiple barriers to overcome in addressing his health issue.

Systematic reviews of evidence in relation to the built and natural environment confirm that it influences physical activity. Specifically, our transport infrastructures, the architectural design of our schools and workplaces, spatial planning of built environments and urban green spaces are identified as having an important influence on people's physical activity (National Institute for Health and Clinical Excellence, 2008). Work by the National Institute for Health and Clinical Excellence (NICE) supports, at least in part, the revised model of health determinants put forward by Barton and Grant (2006).

So a brief consideration of the questions, what do we mean by the term health and what determines health, leads us to a sense that the notion of health is much more than absence of disease and that a wide range of factors with complex interactions influences it. It should be noted that the models of Dahlgren and Whitehead and Barton and Grant do not imply directionality: determinants can be a positive or negative influence on health outcomes.

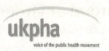

Health Map

A tool for investigating the impacts of the natural and built environment on public health, developed in association with the UKPHA Strategic Interest Group and the World Health Organisation Healthy Cities programme

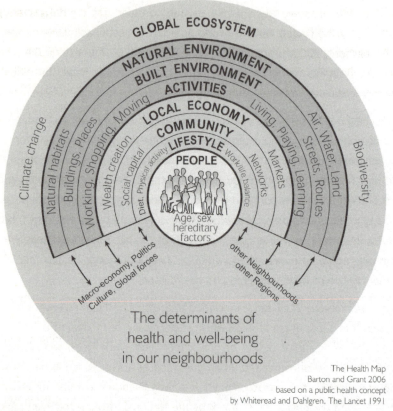

WHO Collaborating Centre for Healthy Cities
Faculty of the Built Environment
University of the West of England
BRISTOL

Figure 3.1 The Health Map

Source: Barton and Grant (2006)

Natural environments and their influence on health

The 'determinants of health and well-being in our neighbourhoods' model indicates that the natural environment and global ecosystem have an important influence on people's health, but is this really the case, in countries like the UK, Italy, Japan or Canada?

The demands of modern urban life can make it seem that the natural environment is something remote and without influence on our lives. People are generally not engaged with nature. Nature is the birds, insects and plants of documentary programmes on television, not part our everyday life. This disengagement leads to a perception that people are not part of the natural world and that it has no influence upon us. In reality we are far closer to nature than we think and this link affects our health.

Human evolution provides an important starting point for considering the natural environment and health. Our evolutionary ancestors *australopithecus* lived approximately 3–4 million years ago. Initially forest dwelling, *australopithecus* evolved into a plain dweller. Then about 2 million years ago it involved into *homo habilis*, a species that lived in a variety of habitats. *Homo sapien sapien* appeared approximately 200,000 years ago, but it is only in the last 10,000 years that human beings have pursued agriculture and developed urban civilizations (Baldia, 2003). For the vast majority of our evolutionary history our ancestors were very much engaged with and shaped by their natural environment. *Homo sapien sapien* has slowly evolved in response to the natural environments and habitats it encountered.

It can be argued that the adaptation and change of our environment over the last 10,000 years (agriculture, urbanization, industrialization) has been too rapid to be accommodated by biological evolutionary processes. In any organism where we observe displacement into alien environments we might expect to see physiological stress, reduced fecundity, increases in the disease burden and mortality rates and, in extremes, local extinction. Given our evolution, are people really different? Can we continue to thrive if the environment to which we are adapted fundamentally and rapidly changes?

In 1984 the Harvard biologist, Edward Wilson, argued through the proposition of the 'biophilia hypothesis': that we really are not that different from other animals. To Wilson it seemed incontrovertible that we have an innate sensitivity to and need for living things, because we have existed in a close relationship with nature for most of our history (Wilson, 1984). The biophilia hypothesis puts a connection or contact with nature at the very core of our health. Van den Berg et al (2007) also recognize the challenges of living in urban environments and the need for contact with nature to maintain psychological health and well-being.

Mitchell and Popham (2008) looked to see if exposure to natural environments affected health inequalities in the working-age population of England. The 'exposure measure' was the proportion of green space in a neighbourhood, represented by lower level super output areas (LSOAs), a unit used for reporting small area statistics in England. Each LSOA was characterized by the proportion of land area classed as green space, by income-deprivation, by all-cause mortality and by three other causes of death. Mitchell and Popham concluded that health inequalities related to income deprivation were reduced in the poorest populations exposed to the greenest environments. A study based in Tokyo, Japan, found that access to walkable green spaces in urban areas increased the longevity of senior citizens (Takano et al, 2002).

As well as the idea that contact with and access to natural environments, even within urban areas, is good for an individual's physical health, the idea that it is also good for a person's mental health has been explored. A study of recreational walkers in the city of Sheffield in England found a positive association between biodiversity and people's 'perception of mood score' (POMS). When people had direct contact with green spaces, which were rich in wildlife, their feelings of anxiety and stress declined more than when they experienced being outside in a 'sports field type' grassland or monotonous municipal park (Fuller et al, 2007).

Studies exposing people to different images whilst exercising, such as a streetscape or a lakeland scene, have also noted a reduction in anxiety and stress associated with the 'natural scene' exposure, as did an experiment exposing people to a shopping mall experience and country walks (Pretty et al, 2006; Pretty, 2007). Hartig et al (1991, 2003) found that contact with nature through the activity of walking had a restorative effect, reducing attention deficits arising from over working and over-concentration when compared to walking in urban streets.

These pieces of research are the tip of the iceberg. There is a substantial body of evidence indicating that people do have positive physical and mental responses to contact with natural environments. While none of it proves Wilson's biophilia hypothesis, the accumulating evidence certainly supports the notion that the human species retains a link with the environments that shaped our development for the greater part of our evolutionary history.

The importance of contact with nature

The principle of contact with nature is an important one. Placing this in the context of the extended health determinants model, direct contact with nature falls within the lifestyle or activities segments on the model (see Figure 3.1). Walking and other forms of direct and deliberate contact with natural environments are almost utilitarian in exploiting the natural environment for a positive health benefit – a dose of nature so to speak. It is important to remember that these types of health benefits are most likely a phenomenon of urbanized developed countries. These are the situations where everyday lifestyles may lead to 'nature deprivation' and where nature is benign: wolves, bears or snakes do not threaten you if you go for a walk in Epping Forest on the outskirts of London.

The natural environment of people is more than the nearby woodland that our children play in, or the meadows and parks frequented by people walking their dogs. The word 'environment' refers to those factors and phenomena external to an organism that influence its survival (Begon et al, 1986). The focus of our attention, our organism, is the person. Our interaction, our ecology, with these factors plays a critical role in determining our health.

These factors or phenomena are the environmental systems that underpin life and the transference of energy on our planet. The weather system is one of the more tangible day-to-day factors with which we interact even at the simple level of deciding what clothing to wear each day. Other systems are less apparent, like the water catchment basin system. In economically developed countries our lifestyles make some of these natural environmental systems seem remote, but our interaction with them does determine our health.

There are many natural environmental systems that influence human health, including atmospheric systems, systems that wear away rocks (such as rivers and glaciers) and biological systems that concern the relationship of plants and animals to their environment (such as the detrital and soil system).

Human activity has altered even these most fundamental environmental systems. People have learnt to harness the power of the environment to provide them with products that enhance quality of life. Mesolithic man was amongst the first to realize the possibilities that harnessing nature could offer, as they cleared the forests to make space for agricultural food production. As a means of producing food, agriculture is efficient in harnessing energy from the primary production, detrital and soil systems.

Ecosystem services and human health

The relationship between humans and natural systems, whereby people use and manage natural resources, is expressed in the concept of 'ecosystem services'. The term 'ecosystem services' does not readily conjure up an image; indeed, as an idea, it can feel vague or remote – what have ecosystems got to do with me? The United Nations Millennium Ecosystem Assessment (MEA) is an initiative reviewing the state of the planet and the effects on future social and economic development. Their widely accepted definition considers that ecosystem services are the processes by which environmental resources are produced and can be utilized by humans. These resources include clean air, water, food and material: they are the resources on which our health and well-being are utterly dependent (MEA, 2005; UNEP, 2007). The Millennium Ecosystem Assessment classified ecosystem services as (see Figure 3.2):

- 'supporting services' such as nutrient cycling;
- 'provisioning services', which includes products like food and fuel;
- 'regulating services', the benefits of which include air and water quality;
- 'cultural services' such as recreation.

Table 3.1 shows a differently expressed and more discrete subset of ecosystem services, for which economists have attempted to put a value on

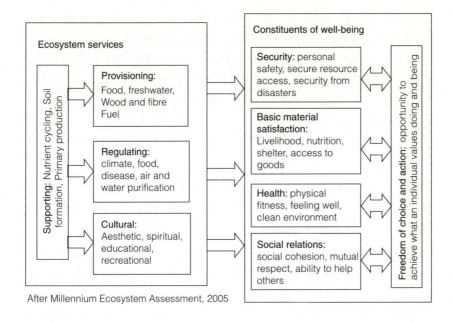

After Millennium Ecosystem Assessment, 2005

Figure 3.2 Ecosystem services and constituents of well-being

Source: MEA (2005)

Table 3.1 Ecosystem services

Global life support services (e.g. oxygen liberation)	*Landscape formation (e.g. coast and river geomorphological processes)*
Flood and erosion control	Waste decomposition and disposal
Water quality and quantity	Pollination
Pollution control	Biological control (e.g. pest reduction)
Soil provision	Habitat provision (e.g. spawning grounds for fish)

Source: Stone (2006)

the environmental products. The values generated by different studies vary substantially, partly because they are looking at outputs that are different in scale from each other and partly because the evaluation methods differ. However, what is generally agreed is that the worth of ecosystem services to humans far outweighs conventional measures of economic wealth like gross domestic product (GDP). In 1997, one estimate placed the annual value of global ecosystem services at US$33 trillion a year, which far exceeded total global economic income (Costanza et al, 1997).

The notion of ecosystems and ecosystem services is an anthropocentric expression of the utilitarian relationship most species have with their natural environments: utility for survival.

It is important to remember that humans are just another animal. For the vast majority of our evolutionary history, we developed in response to the natural environments we encountered. Human ingenuity has enabled us to manipulate our environments to better meet our needs for only a relatively short period in our evolution, and in many parts of the world this environmental manipulation is still limited.

The causal links between human health and environment can be difficult to pin down because they are complex, often indirect and modified by a number of factors. However, ecosystem services and quality natural environments are indispensable to everyone's health and well-being (WHO, 2005b).

As part of the United Nations Millennium Ecosystem Assessment, the WHO produced the report 'Ecosystems and Human Well-being: Health Synthesis' (WHO, 2005b). This report set out a compelling case for the importance of the natural environment and ecosystem services in supporting human health. It also identified the services and products from the environment that underpin our healthy survival.

Water

The first and perhaps most fundamental ecosystem product is fresh water. The provision of fresh water is regulated by the denudation systems, like catchment basins that determine supply, and ecosystems, such as wetlands, that filter water removing potentially toxic elements. Fresh water is essential for human life. In temperate regions, such as the United Kingdom, supplies are usually plentiful and we undervalue it as a resource critical to our survival (WHO, 2005b).

Food

Another essential product for human survival is food, which, in its different shapes and forms, is a resource derived from ecosystems. Agriculture is the utilization and taming of the primary production system (naturally occurring plants and animals) in order to maximize the yield of 'useful resource': food for people. It is still wholly dependent on functional soil and detrital systems and where these start to breakdown, food production is affected. For example, a study of the effect of soil erosion on European crop yields concluded that degradation of the natural system was resulting in productivity losses; it also concluded that erosion-induced productivity declines will become significant in southern European countries in the future, despite the available mechanical and chemical technologies that enable farmers to reduce the immediate impacts (Bakker et al, 2007).

We also get a lot of food from marine ecosystems: shellfish and fish. The marine ecosystem is largely unmanaged and provides vital nutrition for millions of people around the world (WHO, 2005b).

Timber, fibre, fuel, medicines

For many people in the world timber, fibre and fuel are ecosystem products vital to their health and well-being. In economically developed countries the relevance of these products is often lost in pursuit of hi-tech lives, but the dependence remains (WHO, 2005b). Many clothes are made of cotton or wool: cotton comes from a shrub, wool from sheep. Shoes are made of leather: tanned animal hide. We use timber in the construction of our homes. Whilst most of the fuels on which we are dependent, such as gas and oil, are the result of historic ecosystem processes, increasingly biofuels derived from crops and timber are being used to power vehicles and to drive electricity generation.

WHO (2005b) identify the importance of natural products for medicinal purposes. Even today, nearly 80 per cent of people around the world still depend on 'natural' medicinal products (UNEP, 2007). In the developed world most medicines are produced synthetically, but many have natural origins.

Aspirin was derived from the bark of certain species of willow tree (*Salix* spp). The cardio-active drug digitalis was derived from the wayside flower foxglove (*Digitalis purpurea*). The rosy periwinkle (*Catharanus roseus*), a native of the Madagascan rainforests, is the source of two drugs used in the treatment of leukaemia and Hodgkin's Disease: vinblastine and vincristine.

Waste recycling

WHO (2005b) highlight the vital role of ecosystems in breaking down waste and recycling nutrients: processes that contribute to nutritious food, filtered fresh water, even breathable air. The natural environment provides the most fundamental recycling services critical to our health. Ecosystems also give rise to the physical environmental conditions that provide effective barriers to the migration of infectious diseases, particularly when a vector organism is involved, such as mosquitoes transmitting malaria parasites.

The changing environment

Human health is dependent on the natural environment and its ecosystems. This is a complex relationship developed over epochs of interaction, where change has mostly been a gentle evolutionary process. It is also a relationship that operates on different scales, ranging from the large climatic processes that determine the health of whole populations, through to the intimacy of an individual's experience of nearby nature and its mental restorative value (Hartig et al, 1991; Kaplan, 1995). Consequently, the state of the natural environment and ecosystem services is very important for human health.

In 1997, the United Nations Environment Programme (UNEP) established a series of scientific assessments known as the Global Environment Outlook (GEO). These assessments focus on the interactions between the environment and society. The fourth report, produced in 2007, examined the state of and trends in the environment and the human dimensions of the observed change (UNEP, 2007). It is a report that we strongly recommend to all our readers.

Putting climate change to one side (it is considered in detail in Chapter 1), the UNEP GEO 4 assessments report substantial change to the global and local environments that determine our health. The report points to a general deterioration in air quality due to pollution from industrial processes, vehicles, energy generation and large-scale fires. The general decline in air quality is happening despite specific and dramatic improvements in localized urban areas. On the land, GEO 4 raises serious concern about unsustainable use of land and water resources. There is continued soil erosion, nutrition depletion, water scarcity, salinization and chemical contamination of both land and water resources. These factors are influencing the functioning of biological processes and ecosystem services.

Globally, fresh water scarcity is increasing due to excessive groundwater and surface extraction. Deterioration in water quality caused by excessive nutrient loads from land-based activities, such as agriculture, is causing eutrophication (an unhealthy overly rich concentration of nutrients) of inland and coastal water. Pollutants from industrial processes, wastewater and urban run-off further exacerbate the effects of eutrophication, for example causing toxic algal blooms.

The effect of this cumulative pollution on the aquatic and marine environments is to disrupt the ecosystem services. UNEP GEO 4 (2007) also points to the widespread decline of biodiversity and loss of ecosystem services arising from activities like logging of rainforests and drainage of wetlands.

Environmental changes in Europe

Such wholesale changes to the natural environment and ecosystem services are not just a global phenomenon. The GEO 4 report points to worrying environmental trends specific to Europe. These include localized declines in water and air quality, agricultural intensification and land degradation and widespread impacts on landscapes and biodiversity (UNEP, 2007).

Measures of biodiversity in the UK also point to environmental deterioration. Populations of farmland and woodland birds have declined along with those of specialist butterflies, bats and wintering waterbirds. Across the UK the diversity of plants in open habitats, like heaths and grasslands, woodlands and hedgerows, has also declined (JNCC, 2008). These measures are the headline indicators for biodiversity in the UK and are considered to be indicative of underlying natural environment trends. An assessment of the state of the natural environment in England highlighted not only the loss of biodiversity but also particular concerns over the state of the marine environment, the decline in coastal habitats and the deterioration of landscapes, with 20 per cent showing signs of neglect (Natural England, 2008). Urban areas are no exception to this picture of deterioration. There is a declining trend in the UK population of garden birds such as the house sparrow and blackbird (Cannon et al, 2005). The amount of accessible urban green space is also declining as available spaces are sold off to provide land for housing and infrastructure building.

Environmental stress

Our environment is changing! It is changing at global, regional and local levels. Not only is the quantity and quality of our natural environments declining, but the functionality of ecosystem processes is stressed almost to breaking point. The drivers behind this level of environmental change are primarily anthro-pogenic in origin and are often the result of exploitation of natural resources to support unsustainable patterns of consumption (UNEP, 2007). It is antici-pated that anthropogenically driven climate change will increase the rate of environmental change, exacerbating the situation (IPCC, 2007). This will place people everywhere in an increased state of environmental stress, which will have consequences for individual and population health.

The health implications of environmental change

Our degraded natural environments, dysfunctional ecosystem services and climate change will affect everyone's health. The precise impacts on individuals will be modified by location, age, gender and socio-economic status: all the usual determinants of health. The expressions of environmental degradation will also vary spatially and temporally: not all people will be affected in the same way, to the same degree or at the same time. Despite this variability, it is possible to anticipate some of the human health impacts that will be experi-enced if environmental change follows current trajectories.

Climate change

The health impacts of climate change are reviewed in detail in Chapter 2. It is important to note, however, that the damage to health caused by climate change is linked to a breakdown in environmental systems. For example, the consequences of climate change regarding floods, heat waves and vector- and rodent-borne disease represent significant risks to human health (Menne and Ebi, 2006). Each of these health impacts represents a breakdown, at least in part, of natural processes and ecosystem services. For example, shifting climatic zones due to warming are removing the ecological barriers to the distribution of the ticks that are largely responsible for the transmission of Lyme disease. The consequence of environmental degradation is an increased incidence of Lyme disease in northern Europe (Lindgren and Jaenson, 2006).

The case of Lyme disease is illustrative of the anticipated consequences of climatic zone shift, changes in humidity, temperature etc., broadly the change of ecological barriers to species survival. This phenomenon has prompted commentators to point to the possibility of the evolution of new disease vectors and reservoirs, the emergence of new pathogens driven by adaptation to biodiversity loss and range changes of existing vectors such as mosquitoes (Hales et al, 2002; ECDC, 2007; Gage et al, 2008; St. Louis and Hess, 2008).

Water

Water is important to our health. The projected changes in the environment and ecosystem processes are likely to increase localized flooding and droughts and cause disruption of the hydrological cycle. These changes could result in increases in respiratory distress and diarrhoeal disease outbreaks, particularly amongst the most vulnerable in our society (St. Louis and Hess, 2008).

Agriculture

Our agricultural systems are also being stressed by changes in the environment, which also has implications for health. The stresses on agriculture may lead to reductions in food production even in temperate regions of the world. Townsend et al (2003) suggest that the nitrogen cycle may break down, leading to nitrogenous pollution of air and water, which is associated with respiratory ailments, cardiac disease and some cancers. Excess nitrogen in the soil system can also lead to higher production of allergenic pollens. Boxall et al (2008) go further and suggest that changes in the environment, in particular extreme weather events, will increase the likelihood of exposure to agricultural contaminants, both chemical and pathogenic.

Overall impact

Our environment, its underlying processes and its ecosystem services are changing. Anthropogenically driven climate change, exploitation and destruction of natural resources and disruption of natural processes are accelerating the rate of change. Human health is inexorably linked to the natural environment and the degree of change we are already experiencing threatens even the basic requirements for maintaining health: food, shelter, fuel, clean air and water.

Degraded environments are associated with high levels of mortality. Each year 800,000 people die from causes attributable to urban air pollution; 3.2 million from water-borne diseases; 1.8 million from diseases associated with a lack of access to clean water; 3.5 million from malnutrition and 60,000 from natural disasters (WHO, 2005b; 2008). Current environmental trends will only cause these numbers to increase. Environmental mortality will increasingly impact on developed countries, as our complex relationship with the natural world is pushed to breaking point.

Sustainable development

Climate change, dysfunctional ecosystems and degradation of natural resources can no longer simply be considered as environmental or developmental problems. We have seen that the health and well-being of everyone is determined directly and indirectly by our complex relationship with the environment. Delivery of public health goals in the future will increasingly depend on the delivery of environmental goals at local, regional and global levels. This is a reflection of the interdependence that has been described throughout this chapter.

Another part of this equation is economic development. The idea that social justice, environmental care and economic development are interdependent and need to be given equal consideration is the idea of sustainable development. This was codified by the United Nations at the 1992 summit in Rio de Janeiro, though its origins might go as far back as *Silent Spring* (Carson, 1962). (Now recognized as one of the most influential books of the 20th century, *Silent Spring* exposed the destruction of wildlife through the widespread use of pesticides.)

The drive for social justice, heath equality, environmental justice and economic development that do not compromise the chances of future generations, all come together in the aspirations of sustainable development. The concept of sustainable development recognizes that the world is a series of complex inter-actions and interdependencies. Consideration of how to apply the principles in practice gave rise to the Millennium Ecosystem Assessments, described earlier, that identified health and environmental issues as universal priorities to be addressed by all countries (WHO 2005b; UNEP, 2007).

Definition of sustainable development

The most widely used definition of sustainable development is 'development which meets the needs of the present without compromising the ability of future generations to meet their own needs' (World Commission on Environment and Development, 1987). Implicit to this definition of sustainable development and its forward looking vision is the application of the precautionary principle in environmental decision-making, which was made explicit through Principle 15 of the Rio Declaration (UNEP, 1992) Broadly, the precautionary principle is an approach to decision-making that justifies preventive measures or policies despite scientific uncertainty about whether detrimental effects will occur.

The UK has agreed five shared principles for sustainable development (Defra, 2005):

1   Living within environment limits: respecting the limits of the planet's environment, resources and biodiversity; to improve our environment and ensure that the natural resources needed for life are unimpaired and remain so for future generations.
2   Ensuring a strong, healthy and just society: meeting the diverse needs of all people in existing and future communities, promoting personal well-being, social cohesion and inclusion and creating equal opportunity for all.
3   Achieving a sustainable economy: building a strong, stable and sustainable economy that provides prosperity and opportunities for all, and in which environmental and social costs fall on those who impose them (the 'polluter pays' principle) and efficient resource use is incentivized.

4   Using sound science responsibly: ensuring policy is developed and implemented on the basis of strong scientific evidence, whilst taking into account scientific uncertainty (through the Precautionary Principle as well as public attitudes and values.

5   Promoting good governance: actively promoting effective, participative systems of governance at all levels of society; engaging people's creativity, energy and diversity.

The UK's sustainable development strategy (Defra, 2005) identifies four priority themes:

1   Sustainable consumption and production: the principle of living within natural resource constraints and achieving more with what we have, with much less waste.

2   Climate change and energy.

3   Natural resource protection and environmental enhancement, which includes the concept that health and well-being is linked to environmental quality and ecosystem services.

4   Sustainable communities: addressing multiple inequalities and cycles of poverty and degradation.

Sustainable development strategies such as this provide a framework for positive change, including the action suggested in Part II of this book. They present an opportunity for different constituencies, such as health practitioners and environmentalists, to come together to address shared problems with the aim of achieving real joint benefits.

Conclusion

People's health is determined by the natural environment and the ecosystem services it provides. The future health of communities and populations is directly threatened by our destruction and degradation of the very environment that supports our lives. To maintain and enhance people's health, we must nurture our environment through joined-up action that delivers truly sustainable development within the limits of the available natural resources.

'The earth we abuse and the living things we kill will, in the end, take their revenge; for in exploiting their presence we are diminishing our future.' Marya Mannes, *More in Anger*, 1958

References

Bakker M.M., Govers, G., Jones, R.A. and Rounsevell, M.D.A. (2007) 'The effect of soil erosion on Europe's crop yields', *Ecosystems*, vol 10, part 7, pp1209–1219

Baldia, M. (2003) *The Origins of Agriculture* (v2.01), available at www.comp-archaeology.org/AgricultureOrigins.htm (accessed 17 September 2007)

Barton, H. and Grant, M. (2006) 'A health map for the local human habitat', *Journal of the Royal Society for the Promotion of Health*, vol 126, no 6, pp1–2

Begon, M., Harper, J.L. and Townsend, C.R. (1986) *Ecology: Individuals, Populations and Communities*, Blackwell Scientific, Oxford

Boxall, A.B.A., Hardy, A., Beulke, S., Boucard, T., Burgin, L., Falloon, P.D., Haygartg, P.M., Hutchinson, T., Kovats, R.S., Leonardi, G., Levy, L.S., Nichols, G., Parsons, S.A., Potts, L., Stone, D., Topp. E., Turley, D.B., Walsh. K., Wellington, E.M.H.J. and Williams, R.J. (2008) 'Impacts of climate change on indirect human exposure to pathogens and chemicals from agriculture', *Environmental Health Perspectives*, doi: 10.1289/ehp.0800084

Cannon, A.R., Chamberlain, D.E., Toms, M.P., Hatchwell, B.J. and Gaston, K.J. (2005) 'Trends in the use of private gardens by wild birds 1995–2002', *Journal of Applied Ecology*, vol 42, pp659–671

Carson, R. (1962) *Silent Spring*, Houghton Miffin Company, New York

Costanza, R., d'Arge, R., de Groot, R., Farber, S., Grasso, M., Hannon, B., Limburg, K., Naeem, S., O'Neill, R.V., Paruelo, J., Raskin, R.G., Sutton, P. and van den Belt, M. (1997) 'The value of the world's ecosystem services and natural capital', *Nature*, vol. 387, pp253–260

Dahlgren, G. and Whitehead, M. (1991) 'Policies and strategies to promote social equity in health', Institute of Future Studies, Stockholm

Defra (Department for the Environment, Food and Rural Affairs) (2005) 'Securing the Future: the UK Government sustainable development strategy', TSO, London

European Centre for Disease Control (ECDC) (2007) 'Environmental Change and Infectious Disease', Meeting Report, Stockholm 29–30 March 2007, ECDC, Stockholm, Sweden, available at http://ecdc.europa.eu/en/files/pdf/Publications/Environmental_change_and_infectious_disease.pdf

Fuller, R.A., Irvine, K.N., Devine-Wright, P., Warren, P.H. and Gaston, K.J. (2007) 'Psychological benefits of greenspace increase with biodiversity', *Biological Letters*, doi:10.1098/rsbl.2007.0149

Gage, K.L., Burkot, T.R., Eisen, R.J. and Hayes, E.B. (2008) 'Climate and vectorborne diseases', *American Journal of Preventative Medicine*, vol 35, no 5, pp436–450

Hartig, T., Mang, M. and Evans, G.W. (1991) 'Restorative effects of natural environment experiences', *Environment and Behaviour*, vol 23, pp3–26

Hartig, T., Evans, G., Jamner, L.D., Daviss, D.S and Garling, T. (2003) 'Tracking restoration in natural and urban field settings', *Journal of Environmental Psychology*, vol 23, pp109–123

Hales, S., de Wet, N., Maindonald, J. and Woodward, A. (2002) 'Potential effect of population and climate changes on global distribution of dengue fever: an empirical model', *The Lancet*, vol 360, pp830–834

IPCC (2007): 'Climate Change 2007: Synthesis Report', Contribution of Working Groups I, II and III to the Fourth Assessment Report of the Intergovernmental Panel on Climate Change, Pachauri, R.K and Reisinger, A. (eds) (Core Writing Team), IPCC, Geneva, Switzerland

JNCC (2008) *UK Biodiversity Indicators: Overview of Trends*, available at www.jncc.gov.uk/page-4231 (accessed 8 January 2009)

Kaplan, S. (1995) 'The restorative benefits of nature: toward an integrative framework', *Journal of Environmental Psychology*, vol 15, pp169–182

Lindgren, E. and Jaenson, T.G.T (2006) 'Lyme borreliosis in Europe: Influences of climate change, epidemiology, ecology and adaptation measures', in Menne, B. and Ebi, K.L. (eds) *Climate Change and Adaptation Strategies for Human Health*, World Health Organization, Geneva, Switzerland

Mannes, M. (1958) *More in Anger: Some Opinions, Uncensored and Unteleprompted of Marya Mannes*, Lippincott, New York

MEA (2003) 'Ecosystems and human well-being: A framework for assessment', Island Press, London

MEA (2005) 'Ecosystems and human well-being: Current state and trends: findings of the Condition and Trends Working Group', Hassan, R., Scholes, R. and Ash, N. (eds), Island Press, London

Menne, B. and Ebi, K.L. (eds) (2006) *Climate Change and Adaptation Strategies for Human Health*, World Health Organization, Geneva, Switzerland

Mitchell, R. and Popham, F. (2008) 'Effect of exposure to natural environment on health inequalities: an observational population study', *The Lancet*, vol 372, pp1655–1660

National Institute for Health and Clinical Excellence (2008) 'PH8: Physical activity and the environment', National Institute for Health and Clinical Excellence, London

Natural England (2008) *The State of the Natural Environment 2008*, Natural England, Sheffield, UK

Pretty J., Hine R. and Peacock J. (2006) 'Green exercise: the benefits of activities in green places', *The Biologist*, vol 53, no 3, pp143–148

Pretty, J. (2007) *The Earth Only Endures: On Reconnecting With Nature and Our Place in It*, Earthscan, London

St. Louis, M.E., and Hess, J.J. (2008) 'Climate change: impacts on and implications for global health', *American Journal of Preventive Medicine*, vol 35, no 5, pp527–538

Stone, D. (2006) 'Sustainable development: convergence of public health and natural environment agendas, nationally and locally', *Journal of Public Health*, vol 120, pp1110–1113

Takano T., Nakamura, K. and Watanabe, M. (2002) 'Urban residential environments and senior citizens' longevity in megacity areas: the importance of walkable greenspaces', *Journal of Epidemiology and Community Health*, vol 56, no 9, pp13–18

The Information Centre (2008) 'Statistics on obesity, physical activity and diet: England', January 2008, NHS National Statistics

Townsend, A.R, Howarth, R.W., Bazzaz, F.A, Booth, M.S., Cleveland, C.C., Collinge, S.K., Dobson, A.P., Epstein P. R., Holland, E.A., Keeney, D.R., Mallin, M.A., Rogers, C.A., Wayne, P. and Wolfe, A.H. (2003) 'Human health effects of a changing global nitrogen cycle', *Frontiers in Ecology and the Environment*, vol 1, no 5, pp240–246

UNEP (1992) 'United Nations Conference on Environment and Development, Rio, 1992', United Nations Environment Programme

UNEP (2007) 'Global Environment Outlook 4: environment for development', United Nations Environment Programme

Van den Berg, A.E., Hartig, T. and Staats, H. (2007) 'Preference for nature in urbanized societies: stress, restoration, and the pursuit of sustainability', *Journal of Social Issues*, vol 63, no 1, pp79–96

Wilson, E.O. (1984) *Biophilia*, Harvard University Press, Cambridge

World Commission on Environment and Development (1987) 'Our common future', The Brundtland Report, Oxford University Press, Oxford

WHO (2005a) *Basic Documents – 45th Edition*, World Health Organization, Geneva, Switzerland

WHO (2005b) 'Ecosystems and human well-being: Health synthesis', report of the Millennium Ecosystem Assessment, World Health Organization, Geneva

WHO (2008) 'Protecting health from climate change – World Health Day 2008', World Health Organization, Geneva

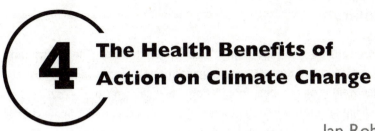

4 The Health Benefits of Action on Climate Change

Ian Roberts

Environmentally friendly policies may feel like a low priority among the many pressures in a busy professional life, but promoting carbon rationing could be your most important contribution to patients' health.

Robin Stott (2006)

Summary

Climate change is a physical sign of a planetary malaise. The Earth's most destructive species (humans) have organized into colonies (economies) and by sheer weight of numbers (population) are damaging the ecosystems on which all life depends. Although there is great interest in how climate change will affect human health much less attention has been paid to the causes of climate change (destructive economies and population growth) and how tackling the underlying causes will affect health. This is unfortunate since there are potentially large benefits for public health through the implementation of policies to prevent further climate change. These policies require an international framework based on equity and justice, such as Contraction and Convergence. Policies to reduce greenhouse gas emissions could bring important reductions in health inequalities, heart disease, cancer, obesity, diabetes, road deaths and injuries and urban air pollution. Reducing animal product consumption in high-income countries is essential to allow increased consumption in poor countries without devastating climate impacts and will bring many health benefits. A rapid transition to a low-energy low-carbon transportation system involving substantially increased levels of active transport, namely walking and cycling, is essential and would also bring with it substantial health benefits: reducing obesity, improving air quality, reducing road deaths and injury and improving mental well-being. Finally, investment in and promotion of family planning could be one of the most cost-effective greenhouse gas reduction measures available, because much of the growth in emissions in coming years will be due to rising population numbers. Some policies to mitigate and adapt to climate change, such as more trees and green spaces, will also improve mental well-being. Promoting human health and equity should be the objective of any humane economic system. Policies to avert climate change have the potential to achieve both of these objectives.

Key terms

Anthropogenic: Pertaining to the effect of human beings on the natural world.

Mitigation: Prevention of further climate change, additional to the changes in the climate that are now inescapable because of the amount of carbon dioxide humankind has already released into the atmosphere.

Contraction and Convergence: A simple, science-based starting point for an international agreement on reducing greenhouse gas emissions proposed by the Global Commons Institute, based on contraction of emissions to an agreed level and convergence by all nations to that level.

Introduction

Two hundred years ago the streets of London were awash with sewage. In 1858 the stench from the river Thames was so strong that MPs declared the House of Commons 'unusable'. Infectious disease was a deadly killer but it was the 'great stink' of 1858 that secured the funds needed to sort out London's sewage (Roberts, 2008). Policy on sewage did more to improve the health of Londoners than any health policy that century. Could responding to climate be the next great health advance?

This chapter argues that putting in place public policies that prevent additional climate change presents unrivalled opportunities for improving public health. As we saw in Chapter 2, climate change and its effect on the ecosystem will have serious implications for health, so preventing runaway climate change is essential for a healthy and sustainable future. However, the economic and social policies that will need to be implemented in order to reduce greenhouse gas emissions will also bring substantial health improvements. Specifically, they could bring important reductions in inequalities in health, heart disease, cancer, obesity, diabetes, road deaths and injuries and urban air pollution.

These health benefits arise for three reasons:

1   Because Contraction and Convergence, which is the fairest, most clearly articulated and most widely supported global framework for

reducing greenhouse gas emissions, has justice and equity at its core and injustice and inequality are major determinants of human suffering and sickness (Global Commons Institute, 2008).

2   Because climate change policies will impact in a health-promoting way on two of the most important determinants of health: human nutrition and human movement.

3   Because climate change policy has to include population policy and the promotion of family planning has huge potential to improve global health (Cleland et al, 2006).

Contraction and Convergence: A policy framework for a stable climate

Contraction and Convergence (C&C) is a simple, science-based starting point for an international agreement on reducing greenhouse gas emissions, based on the principles of justice and equity (Global Commons Institute, 2008). As we saw in Chapter 1, the concentration of greenhouse gases in the atmosphere is increasing. The amount of carbon dioxide, the chief greenhouse gas, is now higher than at any time in the past 650,000 years. To ensure our future survival its concentration must be kept within a safe upper limit. Carbon dioxide remains in the atmosphere for about a century and so in order to keep the atmospheric concentration below a safe limit, the amount of carbon dioxide that is emitted must fall. This is the contraction part. Establishing a safe upper limit is a technical matter for climate scientists, but is likely to be at least an 80 per cent reduction by 2050, maybe more and maybe sooner. Agreement must be reached on where the upper limit should be set and a date by which this concentration should be achieved, and health practitioners need to advocate for this – see Chapter 5 for ideas on how. The question remaining is who should be allowed to emit greenhouse gases?

The atmosphere is a global good that all the citizens of the Earth must take responsibility for and must share. It follows that when it comes to parcelling out entitlement to emit greenhouse gases, everyone should have an equal share. Currently, the emission of greenhouse gases is far from fair. Average per capita carbon emissions of people in the United States are about 20 times higher than that of people in India (see Chapter 1). Contraction and Convergence sets out a timetable for when per capita emissions will converge to equal per capita shares. The policy acknowledges that everyone has an equal right to the atmosphere, but recognizes that the wealthy world will need time to make the transition to fair shares. In the convergence phase, wealthy countries will have to make cuts even as emissions from poorer countries increase; but once per capita emissions converge, rich and poor alike will have to reduce emissions together. The policy also allows for emissions entitlements to be traded, which will again ease the transition to equal shares whilst ensuring that the safe upper limit is not exceeded.

Reducing inequalities

Each year, worldwide, about 10 million children die before their fifth birthday (UN, 2009). They die because they are poor. Poverty condemns them to hunger, dirty water, poor sanitation, inadequate health care, and frequently their parents have had little or no opportunity of education. Contraction and Convergence is a policy response to climate change that simultaneously ensures ecological sustainability and justice for the poor. The carbon profligate will be required to *pay* the carbon thrifty for their unused rights to the atmosphere, thus assuring that the limits of environmental tolerance are not exceeded. In general the rich lead high-carbon lives and the poor lead low-carbon lives, so the policy of C&C should lead to a massive global redistribution of wealth. The lives of African children should not depend on the charitable whims of the wealthy world. C&C ensures that African children's rights to the atmosphere are bought from them rather than stolen.

C&C has the potential to redistribute wealth – and therefore reduce inequalities in health – between countries and within countries. Globally and nationally the carbon greedy would lose out and the carbon frugal would gain. A 2008 study by the UK Department for Environment, Food and Rural Affairs (Defra) found that because low-income households tend to have lower carbon emissions than high-income households, the poorest sections of society would win, whilst the more wealthy sections would lose out (Defra, 2008). When homes are ranked into tenths according to their household income, the Defra study found that 71 per cent of households in the lowest three income tenths would have leftover allowances that they could sell, whilst about half of households in the highest three income tenths would have to buy unused allowances or cut their emissions.

Human nutrition

The impact of food production on climate change

Food production is a significant contributor to the climate change caused by human beings and is estimated to account for one fifth of global greenhouse gas (GHG) emissions. Though the transport of food contributes importantly to the food-related GHG emissions, food production itself is a fossil fuel intensive activity. Indeed, in many respects food is made from oil, or at least consumes a lot of oil in its production. In its daily communion with the sun, the Earth's surface is blessed with about 200 watts of radiant energy per square metre. Plants lift their leaves to receive this radiant energy and after sipping carbon dioxide from the atmosphere, carry out photosynthesis to make the food that sustains life on earth.

For many millennia, sun and soil set limits on the amount of food energy that could be harvested from a given amount of land. However, the availability of seemingly limitless supplies of fossil fuels changed everything. From the 1940s onwards, fossil fuel based fertilizers, pesticides, irrigation and mechanization dramatically increased the amount of food that could be harvested from a given acreage of land.

The contribution of food to climate change and environmental degradation more generally came under particular scrutiny in 2006 following the publication of the report 'Livestock's Long Shadow' by the international Food and Agriculture Organization (FAO). The report identified livestock as being one of the most important contributors to climate change, land degradation, water shortage, water pollution and loss of biodiversity. According to the FAO report, livestock is responsible for about 18 per cent of greenhouse gas emissions when measured in terms of carbon dioxide equivalents.

Land use changes, especially deforestation to provide pasture for grazing, account for the largest share of food-related greenhouse gas emissions. Currently, around one third of the world's land surface is used for livestock, either to provide pasture for grazing or to grow grains for cattle feed. Grain production for feedstock also requires the use of energy-intensive nitrogenous fertilizers. Furthermore, methane released from animal manure and from enteric fermentation is a powerful greenhouse gas with 23 times the global warming potential of carbon dioxide. Livestock is responsible for around 37 per cent of anthropogenic methane emissions. Cattle manure also releases nitrous oxide, a greenhouse gas with nearly 300 times greater global warming potential than carbon dioxide. Livestock accounts for about 65 per cent of anthropogenic nitrous oxide (McMichael et al, 2007).

Global average meat consumption is currently about 100 grams per person per day, ranging from around 25 grams per person in low-income countries to as much as 250 grams per person in high-income countries (McMichael et al, 2007). Increasing population and economic growth are increasing the global demand for meat and milk particularly in East and South Asia and in Latin America. The global production of meat is predicted to more than double between 2000 and 2050 from 229 million tonnes to 465 million tonnes. Milk consumption is also increasing rapidly. These changes will inevitably increase the carbon footprint of livestock even more. Reducing meat and dairy consumption in high-income countries is therefore essential to allow increased consumption in poor countries without devastating climate impacts.

Health benefits of low-carbon diets

The good news for public health is that reducing the consumption of animal products would not only help to stabilize the climate but also, by reducing the amount of saturated fat and meat in the diet, would reduce the incidence of cardiovascular disease and cancer. Saturated fat consumption is the main determinant of blood cholesterol, which is a major cause of cardiovascular disease. Reducing livestock production would reduce saturated fat intake and greatly reduce rates of cardiovascular disease. It could also reduce the incidence of some cancers. The European Code against Cancer (Europe Against Cancer, 2003) recommends a reduction in the intake of foods containing animal fats and an increase in the consumption of fruit and vegetables.

The meat and cancer link is possibly strongest for colorectal cancer with one report estimating that a 100g reduction in daily consumption of red and processed meats would cut the risk of colorectal cancer by about one third (Norat et al, 2005). Colorectal cancer is the second most common cancer in men after lung cancer. It is a cancer that either kills older adults or leaves them having to cope with significant continuing health problems.

The EPIC (European Prospective Investigation into Cancer and Nutrition) diet and cancer study (Norat et al, 2005) was a huge epidemiological research project in which nearly half a million initially cancer free men and women from ten European countries were followed up to assess the link between meat intake and cancer risk. The results showed an association between the consumption of red and processed meats and bowel cancer risk. Among the over 50s, the risk of developing colorectal cancer for those who consumed the smallest quantity of red and processed meat was 1.28 per cent over ten years, compared to 1.71 per cent for those in the highest category of meat intake. A lower risk of breast cancer might also be expected although the extent of the reductions has yet to be properly quantified.

Reducing fatness

Reducing the total quantity of food energy consumed by people in richer countries, particularly the consumption of carbon intensive fats and refined sugar, would also have environmental benefits while reducing the prevalence of fatness, which is now a major health concern worldwide. The association between fossil fuel energy use and fatness operates in both directions. Increased food energy intake, combined with decreased energy output, because in the main we use fossil fuel energy for a lot of our transport, leads to an increase in the prevalence of fatness. Because food production and motorized transport are both energy intensive, they lead to increased greenhouse gas emissions.

However, because more food energy is needed to maintain and move a fat body, fat populations consume more food energy than lean populations. It has been estimated that compared with a 'normal' population (stable mean Body Mass Index – BMI – of about 24), a 'fat' population (stable mean BMI of 29) consumes approximately 208 per cent more food energy.

In other words, the over-consumption of energy (in the form of food) leads to fatness and fatness leads to the over-consumption of energy. Being fat has serious implications for health, increasing the risk of type 2 diabetes, cardio-vascular disease, stroke and some cancers. Tackling fatness by encouraging reduced and healthier food intake and more active transport will therefore benefit both health and the environment.

Human movement: Travel

What sort of world do we want for our children? Enrique Peñalosa, a former Mayor of Bogotá, Colombia (home to 7 million people) found himself considering this question when, after being elected mayor, he was presented with a transportation plan saying that what the city needed was an elevated highway at a cost of $600 million. Peñalosa took a different view:

> We really have to admit that over the past 100 years we have been building cities much more for mobility than for people's well-being. Every year thousands of children are killed by cars. Isn't it time that we build cities that are more child friendly? Over the last 30 years, we have been able to magnify environmental consciousness all over the world. As a result, we know a lot about the ideal environment for a happy whale or a happy mountain gorilla. We are far less clear about what constitutes an ideal environment for a happy human being. One common measure of how clean a mountain stream is to look for trout. If you find the trout, the habitat is healthy. It is the same way with children in a city. Children are a kind of indicator species. If we can build a successful city for children, we will have a successful city for all people.
>
> (Peñalosa and Ives, 2003)

Rather than building the highway, Bogotá installed a high-capacity bus system and created hundreds of pedestrian-only streets, parks, plazas and bike paths. They planted trees and removed ugly signage. Bogotá now boasts the longest pedestrian-only street in the world.

> We chose not to improve streets for the sake of cars, but instead to have wonderful spaces for pedestrians. All this pedestrian infrastructure shows respect for human dignity. We're telling people, 'You are important not because you are rich or because you have a PhD but because you are human.'
>
> (Peñalosa and Ives, 2003)

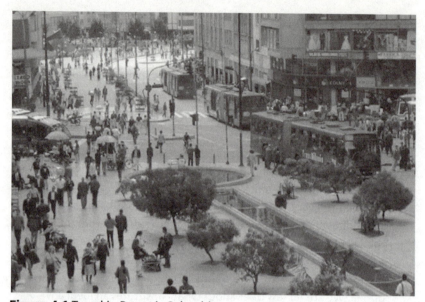

Figure 4.1 Travel in Bogotá, Colombia

Source: www.livablestreets.com/streetswiki/bogota-colombia/bogota_plaza.jpg

Transport, health and climate change

Most urban transportation systems do not respect human dignity nor are they environmentally sustainable. Transportation accounts for about 14 per cent of global greenhouse gas emissions, three quarters of which are from road traffic (Roberts and Arnold, 2007). Transport is the fastest growing source of greenhouse gas emissions in the UK. A rapid transition to a low-energy low-carbon transportation system involving substantially increased levels of active transport, in particular walking and cycling, is essential to avert climate change. Such a strategy would also bring with it substantial health benefits (Roberts and Arnold, 2007).

Road traffic crashes are the leading cause of death for children and young adults in most highly motorized countries. In 2007, approximately 30,000 people were either killed or seriously injured in road traffic crashes in the UK. Worldwide, there are about 1.2 million road deaths each year, with perhaps 10 or 20 times as many people seriously injured. Most of the deaths and injuries are in low- and middle-income countries where numbers are predicted to rise by as much as 80 per cent by 2020 due to increasing motorization (Peden et al, 2004).

Climate change and injury are both partly caused by energy use. Roads can be seen as dangerous rivers of kinetic energy, the energy being derived from the burning of fossil fuels, which leads to the carbon dioxide emissions responsible for climate change. Indeed, the incidence of road traffic injuries has been shown to be a function of fossil fuel energy use by the transportation sector.

Dramatically reducing transportation energy use, by encouraging a modal shift from car use to walking and cycling for short journeys and public transport for longer journeys, will make our streets safer as well as helping to tackle climate change. One study has estimated that had transportation fossil fuel consumption in the USA been cut by 7 per cent in 1990 (the reduction that would have been required under the Kyoto Protocol, see 'key terms' in Chapter 1, assuming the same reduction across all sectors) there would have been 80,000 fewer road deaths in the US between 1990 and 2003 (Roberts and Arnold, 2007).

The road user group who have most to gain from efforts to reduce the volume and speed of road traffic would be pedestrians and child pedestrians in particular. Pedestrian injury is the leading cause of death in children in the UK and it has been demonstrated that injury is linked to social class (Edwards et al, 2006). Pedestrian death rates for children in the poorest social groups are five times higher than those in the most affluent. The most likely reasons for these socio-economic differences is that poor children walk more and they live in more dangerous urban traffic environments than do children from wealthier backgrounds.

Studies consistently show that the volume and speed of traffic is the main environmental determinant of child pedestrian injury risk (Roberts et al, 1995a; Roberts et al, 1995b) The data from case control studies is consistent with the observation that during the 1973 and 1979 oil crises: when traffic volumes and speeds were reduced in an effort to reduce transportation oil use, there were substantial reductions in child pedestrian deaths (Roberts et al, 1992; Roberts and Crombie, 1995).

More recently, mathematical models of pedestrian–motor vehicle collisions have been developed in order to evaluate the effect of transport policies on pedestrian injury risk. The models show that for the same percentage reductions in traffic speed and volume, the largest reductions in injury rates would be from reductions in speed. Pedestrian injury reductions were found to be non-linearly related to traffic speed but linearly related to traffic volume. Apart from limiting the volume and speed of traffic, lowering vehicle mass would also reduce fossil fuel energy use by the transportation sector. The results suggest that this would shift the distribution of casualties towards less severe injuries (Chalabi et al, 2008).

Replacing urban car use by walking, cycling and public transport would reduce fossil fuel energy use thereby mitigating climate change, and by reducing the amount of traffic it would also reduce urban air pollution. Worldwide, urban air pollution – much of which is transport-related – causes about 800,000 premature deaths each year (Woodcock et al, 2007). The introduction of a congestion charge in only a small part of central London has led to modest reductions in levels of nitrogen dioxide and fine particulate matter across the Greater London region, with corresponding increases in life expectancy (Tonne et al, 2008). Increased walking and cycling, by increasing physical activity, would tackle the output side of the personal energy balance equation, helping to reduce the extent of obesity and also the risk of developing some forms of cancer. It would also improve mental well-being.

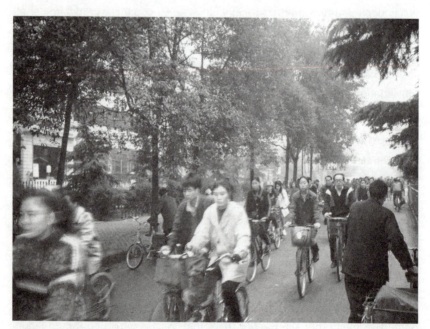

Figure 4.2 China: Cycling as mass transportation

Source: Ian Roberts

Family planning for a sustainable planet

Investment in and promotion of family planning could be one of the most effective greenhouse gas reduction measures available.

Stabilizing global greenhouse gas emissions will be far more difficult in a world of 12 billion people than a world of 8 billion people. Indeed, it has been estimated that 50 per cent of the growth in global carbon dioxide emissions between 1985 and 2025 will have been due to increases in population (Haines et al, 2007). Moreover, per capita emissions of greenhouse gases is rising in many low- and middle-income countries and it is expected that over the coming century 'developing' rather than 'developed' countries will be responsible for most of the growth in greenhouse gas emissions. Policy on population is policy on climate.

The promotion of family planning would have important beneficial effects in terms of reducing greenhouse gas emissions and environmental sustainability, but should also reduce poverty, hunger and deaths of mothers and children. Population growth in poor countries will inevitably increase the number of poor people in the world. In sub-Saharan Africa, population growth made an important contribution to increasing the number of people living on less than a dollar per day from 164 million in 1981 to 316 million in 2001 (Cleland et al, 2006). A large family is a risk factor for family poverty and children from large families are less well-fed and educated than those from smaller families.

Family planning, by increasing the interval between births, is also one of the most cost-effective ways to reduce infant and child mortality. A longer interval between births reduces the risk of foetal death, low birth weight and prematurity. It has been estimated that in 2000, around 90 per cent of abortion-related deaths and 20 per cent of obstetric mortality could have been avoided through the use of family planning methods by women wanting to either postpone or cease having any more children (Cleland et al, 2006).

'Freedom from the tyranny of excessive fertility' (Baird, 1965) would also have important implications for gender equity, human rights and female education. Female education and population control are almost certainly linked in both directions. Improving access to family planning and contraception in order to improve health and well-being, and also to reduce the pressure on the planet's natural resources from the growing population, is a global public health imperative. We are all the inhabitants of a small planet that is facing an unprecedented environmental crisis. Financing family planning in poor countries must become a responsibility of the wealthy world, along with reducing poverty and improving education and health care.

Mental health

This chapter has mainly been concerned with the physical health benefits of action to mitigate climate change. But there is some evidence that reducing greenhouse gas emissions could have mental health benefits as well. Mental well-being should improve:

- Because we will take more physical exercise as a result of reducing our dependence on high-carbon motorized forms of transport, as discussed earlier, and physical exercise is known to promote mental well-being.
- Through the action we will take to improve the quality of the urban environment and provide more green space.
- From reducing levels of material consumption, at least for some,

There is wide-ranging evidence (reviewed by National Heart Forum, 2007; Bird, 2007) that a well-designed urban environment and contact with the natural environment (in some cases even simply being able to have a view of trees) improves our mood, increases social contact, contributes to children's well-being and development and assists patient recovery in health services. As we improve the quality of the built environment – by reducing the volume of motor traffic, providing more and better green space and planting more trees to both mitigate and adapt to climate change (see Chapter 6) – our mental well-being should improve.

More controversially, but worth mentioning if only to stimulate debate, is the relationship between material consumption and mental well-being in richer countries. Consumption of goods and services, other than food, accounts for a quarter of carbon emissions per person in the UK. Even in a time of economic recession, a significant proportion of the population live fairly affluent lives. There is some evidence of a relationship between high levels of material consumption and loss of well-being, such as emotional distress and a feeling of dissatisfaction (see Porritt, 2007; Jackson, 2008 for discussion and references). Therefore a more balanced life that invests more in personal relationships and the community and less in unnecessary material goods is likely to improve mental well-being. In order to de-carbonize and achieve sustainability, the economies of high-income countries will almost certainly have to stabilize, over time, at a lower level of production and consumption of material goods, and invest more in services – as well as making substantial redistributions of income and wealth to reduce social and health inequalities.

The responsibilities of health practitioners

Although the health benefits of action to reduce greenhouse gas emissions are increasingly recognized by health practitioners, they are not yet widely appreciated by those responsible for climate change policy. The purpose of a sustainable human economy should be to promote the health and welfare of all humankind rather than the enrichment of a small percentage. Health practitioners have a responsibility to future generations to ensure that the health benefits of environmental policies are recognized and quantified and that this information is disseminated to our patients, to the public and to policy-makers. Failure to do so would be a serious neglect of our collective responsibility. Part II of this book will offer you a huge range of ideas on how you can play your part – and it is a very important and influential part.

Two for the price of one: Essential synergies in tackling fatness and climate change across the world

Statement from the National Heart Forum, a leading alliance of over 60 national organizations in the UK working to reduce the risk of coronary heart disease and related conditions such as stroke, diabetes and cancer, and a sponsor of this book.

At the time of the publication of the United Kingdom (UK) Foresight Report, *Tackling Obesities Future Choices*, in 2007, Alan Johnson, the UK's Secretary of State for Health, highlighted the scientific study's comparison of the challenge of obesity and climate change. The strategies for addressing both issues share some important features.

Few, even among the medical and health professions, have a clear sense of how the impact of global warming will register for most people, either in the developing countries already prone to rising sea levels, severe weather effects and food insecurity, or among the developed or westernized economies, whose profligacy with the world's finite resources have set us upon a trajectory towards climatic cataclysm that we must avert.

Few, even after Foresight's gloomy prognosis for the UK, have any real sense of how rising levels of obesity, poor-quality diets and activity, not confined to westernized cultures but increasingly widespread across most of the developing world, will impact on our limited capacities for coping with chronic disease, nor how the confounding effects of diminishing agricultural capacity and population movements on an unprecedented scale will further increase the health challenge.

As any reader of this book will have grasped, there are many factors in common. The era of industrialization brought with it not only the pollution and emissions that are implicated in global warming, but a fundamental transformation of our social model, with urbanization altering irrevocably the way in which most of us work and live that is implicated in increasing obesity and related diseases.

More than 50 per cent of the world's population has now become 'urbanized', dependent on an industrialized food supply chain, which is implicated in both the rapid evolution of the obesity epidemic and in climate change. Energy and water-intensive global production to supply sugar and oil, both for human consumption and more recently as bio-fuel, along with corn and cattle, have resulted in the dominance of vast monocultures; in turn this has led to a concentration of cheap components of food production and a preponderance of cost-cutting junk food that tilts the balance against greater dietary variety of choice.

For many, rapid urban concentration has brought a dislocation from traditional diets and from ready access to fresh food. Successive generations have become conditioned to accept a diet composed of largely processed and preserved foods. We are also accustomed to finding products readily available from almost any part of the planet with little thought given to the real cost in energy, emissions, water, labour and the contribution to climate change.

The consequences of climate change will mean that the agricultural land available to feed a future global population of 8 billion people or more is likely to be drastically diminished, and the productive yields of the remaining land may be reduced by higher levels of ultraviolet radiation and crop diseases. We will need to make wiser and more health-efficient use of the land than agribusiness and market forces have dictated up to now; time is short to plan, approve and implement the necessary radical changes to achieve levels of sustainable development that will both feed the world's enlarged population and reduce emissions to help stabilize the rise in global warming.

Global food security presents an immediate and increasing crisis, recognized by the formation of the United Nation's General Secretary's Task Force, but the situation is certain to be exacerbated as the effects of climate change worsen. The political implications are unpredictable, but could be far reaching as climate refugee populations, measured not in tens but hundreds of millions, look to the rest of the world for permanent relocation.

What can be done to support sustainable development and strive towards some measure of stabilization of global warming, which may be the only hope of averting the tipping point when climate change accelerates out of control? Can the demands for improved diets and physical activity levels offer some synergy in applying strategies to cut our energy needs and harmful emissions?

At present in spite of, or perhaps because of, the globalized supply chain which stores and transfers produce via giant supermarket networks, we are often denied the rich local variety of fruit and vegetables brought fresh to market; instead we have become conditioned to insipid substitutes, sometimes of lower nutritional quality, selected primarily for ease of growing and shelf life and transported at high energy cost across continents. This effect is not confined to urban cultures, even tiny populations on Pacific islands have fallen prey, dependent significantly on imported food products, which have displaced indigenous fresh food production. It is no coincidence that South Sea islands such as Samoa, Nauru and Tonga have some of the highest obesity and diabetes rates in the world.

The strategy of sourcing fresh local supplies – something both public and private sector can easily adopt without the need for cumbersome or compelling regulation – is gaining support and has many attractions. It can cut food miles and reduce energy consumption, it may stimulate growth and diversity within the local farming economy, it may to help conserve some of the local varieties of fruit and vegetables squeezed out of mass markets and hopefully it may also revive jaded palates with the flavour of fresher locally grown produce. It is less certain whether 'home grown' food production can wean us away from our global dependence, on any scale that can influence significantly either the dietary changes needed to combat obesity or the energy reductions to combat climate change, but it is an essential step in the right direction.

Our social norms for transport also contribute both to climate change and to reducing the levels of physical activity needed to maintain a healthy weight and reduce the risk of cardiovascular diseases, diabetes and some cancers. The dense urban environments that impair access to healthier food also impair access to activity. Contributing to combating climate change by reducing our use of cars can lead to a reciprocal benefit with more people cycling or walking. However we must recognize that mass air travel – whatever the incentives – remains one of the major contributors to climate change, an even more significant challenge still largely overlooked.

Health practitioners around the world face a daunting set of challenges. Rising temperatures may bring sharp reversals in the attempts to eradicate malaria and other communicable diseases may become a greater threat. An increase in the incidence of heart attacks and stroke is feared as heat waves become more frequent. Already rising food prices, compounded by climate-induced reductions in agricultural productivity, may lead to a continuation of the global obesity trends with even greater dependence on cheaper calorie-dense nutrient-poor foods with healthier diets becoming even less affordable.

However it is encouraging that in the UK, the National Health Service is demonstrating 'corporate leadership' in addressing climate change. If it were a country, the NHS would rank as the 30th largest global economy with a £90 billion annual budget. As the largest public sector contributor to climate change in the UK, it is responsible for 18 million tonnes of carbon dioxide emissions each year, and therefore has enormous potential to seek and signpost the strategic changes that others might adopt. In partnership with others, it has established its own Sustainable Development Unit and has adopted strategies to look at ways to cut food miles, to stimulate procurement of local fresh produce and cut its energy consumption (see Chapter 11).

It is but one example to show that the health sector can and must play an influential role in leading the way forward.

Source: Neville Rigby and Paul Lincoln

References

Baird, D. (1965) 'A fifth freedom?' *British Medical Journal*, vol 2, pp1141–1148

Bird, W. (2007) 'Natural Thinking – Investigating the Links between the Natural Environment, Biodiversity and Mental Health', RSPB, available at www.rspb.org.uk/Images/naturalthinking_tcm9-161856.pdf (accessed 8 February 2009)

Chalabi, Z., Roberts, I., Edwards, P. and Dowie, J. (2008) 'Traffic and the risk of vehicle-related pedestrian injury: a decision analytic support tool', *Injury Prevention*, vol 14, pp196–201

Cleland, J., Bernsatein, S., Ezeh, A., Faundes, A., Glasier, A. and Innis, J. (2006) 'Family planning: the unfinished agenda', *The Lancet*, vol 368, pp1810–1827

Defra (2008) 'Personal Carbon Trading', available at www.defra.gov.uk/environment/climatechange/uk/individual/carbontrading/index.htm (accessed 9 February 2009)

Edwards, P., Roberts, I., Green, J. and Lutchman, S. (2006) 'Deaths from injury in children and employment status in family: analysis of trends in class specific death rates', *British Medical Journal*, vol 333, p119

Europe Against Cancer (2003) 'European Code Against Cancer and Scientific Justification', 3rd version, European Union, available at www.cancercode.org (accessed 8 February 2009)

Food and Agricultural Organization (2006) *Livestock's Long Shadow: Environmental Issues and Options*, Food and Agricultural Organization, Rome

Global Commons Institute (n.d.), available at www.gci.org.uk/ (accessed 8 February 2009)

Government Office for Science and Innovation (2007) 'Foresight – Tackling Obesities – Future Choices', available at www.foresight.gov.uk/OurWork/ActiveProjects/Obesity/KeyInfo/Index.asp (accessed 8 June 2009)

Haines, A., Smith, K.R., Anderson, D., Epstein, P.R., McMichael, A.J., Roberts, I., Wilkinson, P., Woodcock, J. and Woods, J. (2007) 'Policies for accelerating access to clean energy, improving health, advancing development, and mitigating climate change', *The Lancet*, vol 370, no 9594, pp1264–1281

Jackson T (2008) 'The Challenge of Sustainable Lifestyles', Chapter 4 in The Worldwatch Institute, *State of the World 2008: Innovations for a Sustainable Economy,* Worldwatch Institute, Washington, DC

McMichael, A.J., Powles, J.W., Butler, C.D. and Uauy, R. (2007) 'Food, livestock production, energy, climate change, and health', *The Lancet*, vol 370, pp1253–1263

National Heart Forum, Living Streets, CABE (2007) *Building Health. Creating and Enhancing Places for Healthy, active lives*, National Heart Forum, London

Norat, T., Bingham, S., Ferrari, P. et al (2005) 'Meat, fish, and colorectal cancer risk: the European prospective investigation into cancer and nutrition', *Journal of the National Cancer Institute*, vol 97, pp906–916

Peden, M., Scurfield, R., Sleet, D. et al (2004) 'World Report on Road Traffic Injury Prevention', World Health Organization, Geneva

Peñalosa, E. and Ives, S. (2003) 'The Politics of Happiness', available at www. yesmagazine.org/article.asp?ID=615 (accessed 11 February 2009)

Porritt, J. (2007) *Capitalism as if the World Matters* (revised edition) Earthscan, London

Roberts, I., Marshall, R. and Norton, R. (1992) 'Child pedestrian mortality and traffic volume in New Zealand', *British Medical Journal*, vol 305, p283

Roberts, I., Norton, R., Jackson, R., Dunn, R. and Hassall, I. (1995a) 'Effect of environmental factors on risk of injury of child pedestrians by motor vehicles: a case-control study', *British Medical Journal*, vol 310, pp91–94

Roberts, I., Marshall, R. and Lee-Joe, T. (1995b) 'The urban traffic environment and the risk of child pedestrian injury: a case-crossover approach', *Epidemiology*, vol 6, pp169–171

Roberts, I. and Crombie, I. (1995) 'Child pedestrian deaths: sensitivity to traffic volume – evidence from the USA', *Journal of Epidemiology and Community Health*, vol 49, pp186–188

Roberts, I. (2007) 'Comment and analysis: say no to global guzzling', *New Scientist*, June, vol 309, p21

Roberts, I. and Arnold, E. (2007) 'Policy at the crossroads: climate change and injury control', *Injury Prevention*, vol 13, no 4, pp 222–223

Roberts, I. (2008) 'The economics of tackling climate change', *British Medical Journal,* vol 336, pp165–166

Stott, R. (2006) 'Healthy response to climate change', *British Medical Journal*, vol 332, pp1385–1387

Tonne, C., Beevers, S., Armstrong, B., Kelly, F. and Wilkinson, P. (2008) 'Air pollution and mortality benefits of the London Congestion Charge: spatial and socioeconomic inequalities', *Occupational and Environmental Medicine*, available at http://oem.bmj.com/cgi/content/short/oem.2007.036533v1 (accessed 8 June 2009)

UN (2009) www.un.org/millenniumgoals (accessed 9 February 2009)

Woodcock, J., Banister, D., Edwards, P., Prentice, A.M. and Roberts, I. (2007) 'Energy and transport', *The Lancet*, vol 370, no 9592, pp1078–1088

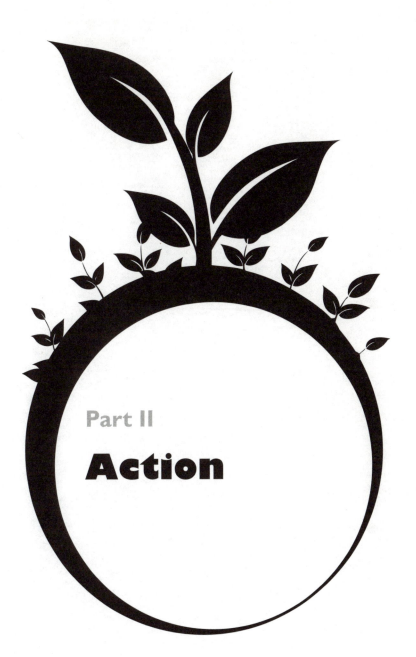

Part II

Action

Introduction to Part II

Fiona Adshead

> The more we study the major problems of our time, the more we come to realize that they cannot be viewed in isolation. They are systemic problems, which means that they are interconnected and interdependent.
>
> Fritjof Capra, *The Web of Life* (1996)

Throughout this book, we demonstrate the clear definition of the links between climate change and health. We argue that change really is possible wherever and whenever we live, work and play – and that everybody in society has a part to play. We recognize the critical role of national and local government and international agencies. Their roles have constraints because governments have to balance and act on a range of competing interests, which are increasingly global. The financial crisis of 2008 and 2009 demonstrated how fragile global systems can be, but the interdependence and interconnectedness of countries' economies have also offered new opportunities for leadership and shown that governments can choose, if they wish, to implement solutions that previously seemed improbable. Influencing governments in the face of these pressures can be quite a challenge – but as Part II of the book suggests, there are many ways in which health practitioners can influence change at national and international levels through our everyday practice and through joining with others to advocate collectively.

As you work your way through the chapters in Part II, you will find many examples of ways in which we are already having an impact through our daily work, by reinforcing the connections between health and climate change and contributing to the more effective implementation of public health, sustainable development and environmental policies. We hope Part II will help you to find the tools to enable such action to become the norm, rather than still relatively isolated examples of good practice.

But where should we start? A good way in is to go back to the basic and fundamental principles of public health.

1 Use sound science responsibly

'A great deal more discipline is needed to ensure that problems are clearly identified and tackled, that the multiple solutions frequently needed are sensibly co-ordinated and that lessons are learnt which feed back directly into policy'. HM Treasury, 2004.

Chapter 2 in Part I described how the health impacts of climate change are already manifesting themselves around the world – making the case for a step change in the way in which we practice. We need to draw upon the considerable evidence base available to direct our practice, some of which is highlighted in the chapters that follow. At all levels, local, national and international, there is an urgent need for a coherent strategy for collecting, interpreting and disseminating this evidence base, building on the research, learning and guidance-producing networks that exist in many countries, which need to give a high priority to mitigation and adaptation to climate change and related environmental issues.

We need to identify common solutions to complex social problems and act decisively if we are to achieve the level of change that is required. This means recognizing and capitalizing on the interactions between settings to maximize our impact (see Figure II.1).

Throughout Part II of this book we have incorporated guidance and examples on the use of a range of specific systems, tools and ideas that we believe may be valuable to health practitioners in addressing the challenges of radically reducing greenhouse gas emissions and adaptation to climate change. The resources section at the end provides a selection of websites of organizations and groups to give you more information, ideas and support, and also some sources of further information on key issues ranging from energy and health to preventing and coping with floods.

But, fundamentally, we want you to feel empowered to fulfil your own potential, so that the complex behavioural challenges associated with action on climate change are recognized as shared challenges that we face together as a

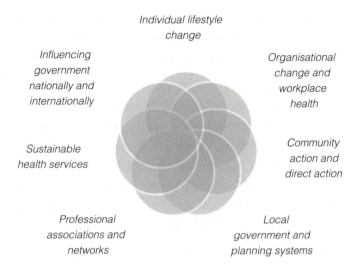

Individual lifestyle
change

Influencing
government
nationally and
internationally

Organisational
change and
workplace
health

Sustainable
health services

Community
action and
direct action

Professional
associations and
networks

Local
government and
planning systems

Figure II.1 Interactions between settings

community. This is not just about our personal roles in addressing single issues, it is also about recognizing common causes and common solutions that span issues – and then acting creatively and in partnership with others to address them.

2 Frame issues so that collective responses are facilitated

Action in one setting will almost certainly lead naturally, over time, into action in another setting. As we engage with climate change and health in all aspects of our life and work, we will motivate others to take similar action simply through our day-to-day interaction with them.

But this is not enough. Increasingly, as our knowledge of systems and experience of partnership working evolves, we are becoming more aware of the complex web of interlinkages between policy and thematic areas. Public health experts have written extensively on frameworks that offer solutions to working across boundaries – from simple partnerships to 'ecological' models. There is a growing and robust library to draw upon, nationally and internationally. The value of this broad partnership approach is emphasized, for example, in

Chapter 5 on leadership to influence national and international policy, Chapter 6 on helping to plan sustainable communities, Chapter 9 on taking action in the community and Chapter 10 on helping organizations to take action.

The concept of 'syndemic orientation', which means an explicit focus on the connections between health problems and their shared origins, offers a broader framework for considering health problems and addressing the dynamic inter-actions between them. It promotes a proactive systemic approach that actively explores the connections between complex problems and, having identified their common root causes, suggests partnership approaches to secure the synergistic solutions that cannot be achieved in isolation. This approach could be fundamental to our approach to tackling climate change.

An example of 'syndemics' is the interaction between the obesity epidemic in high-income countries and climate change, which is repeatedly referred to in this book. Obesity is a symptom of unsustainable development. Its causes, such as dependence on the car and inappropriate food consumption, are also causes of climate change and the wider environmental crisis. The solutions lie in a 'bold whole system approach', a set of integrated policies from the produc-tion and promotion of health diets, to redesigning the built environment to promote walking, together with wider cultural changes to shift societal values around food and activity (Government Office for Science, 2007).

3 Lead by example

Several chapters identify the key role that government can play. But policies alone are not enough – they set a direction and act as a catalyst for action. A catalyst speeds up the rate of change, but depends on active leadership to coalesce and motivate stakeholders so that they not only recognize a common purpose, but are motivated to drive forward the agenda. Building commitment amongst autonomous professionals and gaining their support is a recognized skill of the health professional. The involvement of clinicians in management has been shown to be crucially important in achieving and sustaining change across health services (Joss and Kogan, 1995). Driving forward action on climate change has to be recognized as a shared priority. As health practitioners, we are uniquely placed to play a key role, leading both by example and engaging the right partners to enable others in our local communities to take effective action too.

4 Look for common causes and risks across policy and practice areas and then work in partnership to exploit opportunities for dual delivery

There are many examples of the interdependence of the climate change and health agendas. Chapter 6 shows how sustainable transport policies, for example, can contribute both to our collective action on climate change by reducing carbon emissions, but also to tackling obesity and other chronic diseases by promoting physical activity. This recognition underpins much national policy. But arguably, it is not translating effectively into widespread, commonplace action on the ground. Why?

As you will be well aware, effective implementation in communities has often been very difficult. The traditional approach of health practitioners has often focused on one disease or risk factor at a time, such as diabetes or smoking. Whilst we may recognize that there are shared social, biological, environmental and behavioural factors across policy areas, our recognition has not necessarily translated into a shared, coherent approach to addressing such factors across policy and practice silos.

Health practitioners have long recognized that working in silos, as independent professional tribes each with their own turf, is not conducive to achieving health outcomes. Successful partnership in practice has been demonstrated to achieve improved outcomes, by focusing on the benefits of working together on such complex issues as obesity and teenage pregnancy to achieve shared and speci-fied outcomes. The risks of failure are too great to limit our action by failing to cluster the risk factors, interdependencies and collective attributes effectively, and using this information to develop and inform coherent strategies. If we want to maximize our potential impact, we need to challenge ourselves, as well as challenge others. This book, and Part II in particular, argues that to avert catastrophic climate change we cannot afford such a fragmented approach if we are to act in time. Each chapter suggests solutions that are powerful precisely because they bring together a complex network of policy areas.

5 Communicate effectively with ourselves and with potential partners – ensuring our messages appeal to our target audience encouraging them to act

Promoting personal action on climate change has to fit in with other aspects of people's lives, their lifestyles and aspirations. As Chapters 7 and 11 in particular describe, living within the limited availability of natural resources on a daily basis is directly linked to health outcomes and more fundamentally to the sustainability of health care systems. This book gives many examples of work at a local level that builds on this understanding of the perspectives of different partners and communities to provide real solutions. So we know that things are already happening – but we need to sustain this change and accelerate the process, so that such examples become the norm.

If the relationships between health and climate change are complex, so too are the relationships between leadership, the state, the individual and community action. By illustrating the congruence between their agendas, Part II provides a sound platform for harnessing the power and leadership potential of health practitioners to spread ideas and promote meaningful action across society.

We need to learn from our past, recognize the consequences of our actions and act now to protect our future. As Martin Luther King Jr (1967) so eloquently said:

> We are now faced with the fact that tomorrow is today. We are confronted with the fierce urgency of now. In this unfolding conundrum of life and history there is such a thing as being too late... We may cry out desperately for time to pause in her passage, but time is deaf to every plea and rushes on. Over the bleached bones and jumbled residue of numerous civilizations are written the pathetic words: 'Too late'.

We hope Part II will help you to ensure that in the case of action to combat climate change, our collective epitaph is not 'too little, too late...'.

References

Capra, F. (1996) *The Web of Life*, Anchor Books, New York

Government Office for Science (2007) 'Foresight: Tackling Obesities: Future Choices', available at www.foresight.gov.uk/OurWork/ActiveProjects/Obesity/Obesity.asp (accessed 4 March 2009)

HM Treasury (2004) 'Securing Good Health for the Whole Population' (the Wanless Report), HMT, London

Joss, R. and Kogan, M. (1995) *Advancing Quality*, Open University Press, Buckingham

Martin Luther King Jr (1967) 'Beyond Vietnam', address delivered to the clergy and laymen concerned about Vietnam at Riverside Church, 4 April, New York City

5 Leadership: How to Influence National and International Policy

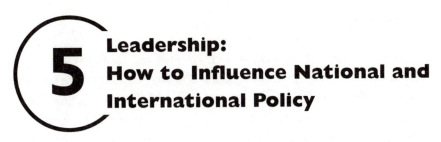

Mike Gill and Robin Stott

If not us, who; if not now, when?

Rabbi Hillel,
from the Talmud, and attributed to Robert F. Kennedy

Summary

Health practitioners have a crucial and distinctive role to play in influencing public opinion and the policies of national and international governments and agencies. Through their numbers and the reach of their influence, health practitioners can play a key part in triggering collective shifts in public consciousness and support for action. They can argue powerfully that much of what we should be doing to mitigate climate change, we should be doing anyway for good public health reasons. We must use the trust of the public and the weight of scientific evidence. We must inform, affirm, advocate, innovate and disseminate, focusing our efforts on the implementation of a global framework that requires a major reduction in carbon emissions from the rich world and, within an overall reducing amount of carbon emissions, enables a rise in emissions for the poor world to assist their development. We need to understand and use effectively the processes that exert pressure on governments to change, for example the United Nations, the European Union and the World Health Organization, and domestically the roles of government departments, non-governmental organizations and citizen groups. We need to learn from the past, for example the control of tobacco, how to overcome 'the manufacture of uncertainty'. We need to work with and support other like-minded groups to develop a global social movement.

Key terms

Advocacy: To generate the legitimizing momentum to allow governments to feel safe and emboldened to take the right action.

United Nations Framework Convention on Climate Change: Annual conferences to produce international agreements to reduce greenhouse gas emissions. The Kyoto Protocol will be replaced by targets agreed in Copenhagen in December 2009.

Non-violent direct action: Often inspired by Gandhi's ideas of Satyagraha or 'truth force', it is characterized by Martin Luther King as 'action which seeks to create such a crisis and foster such a tension that a community which has constantly refused to negotiate is forced to confront the issue. It seeks so to dramatize the issue that it can no longer be ignored'.

Introduction

A key aim of this book is to ensure that health arguments are deployed more effectively to make change happen. In this chapter we focus on how health practitioners can make a real impact on the action of governments nationally and internationally to tackle climate change. We set out what is distinctive about our contribution and propose how we might best make that contribution. If the planet is to continue to be habitable, the scale of reduction in global greenhouse gas emissions required is so urgent and so large that:

- Technological developments can play a part, but only a part, in achieving this reduction.
- Very significant behaviour change is required by individuals, organizations (including health services and local government) and communities – and later chapters will offer you many ideas on how you can make a real difference.
- This change can admit no 'refuseniks' since they would place yet more burden of reduction of greenhouse gas emissions on the rest of us and the adequacy of our collective action would be threatened.

121

- Agreement is therefore required on an international, indeed global, scale not just to cap emissions, but also on mechanisms for implementing this cap.

Governments tend to be constitutionally cautious. When they are not, it is because they feel secure that they will not lose the support of their electorates. The best recent example of this was the intervention by governments to deal with the global banking crisis in 2008. For the electorate in almost all countries affected the choice was between supporting the bold action by the government to reduce the risk of losing their job, their pension and in some cases their home, or being certain to do so. Niceties of political ideology played second fiddle, even in the US.

The acuteness of the climate crisis is yet to occupy the same space in the minds of most electorates as the financial and subsequent economic crisis. Dominant patterns of culture, business and politics still generally serve to maintain climate change: its reality has not yet struck home. That is why we are still largely in the phase of fine rhetoric about brave intentions. We are not yet seeing governments take action on the required scale. In such circumstances the job of citizens must be to help governments feel not just able, but compelled, to take the necessary action. A main argument of this chapter is that health practitioners are peculiarly well placed to provide such help.

Health practitioners have a distinctive part to play in advocating the radical policies required to tackle adequately the major issues faced by 21st century-mankind. The aim of advocacy in this context is to generate the legitimizing momentum that allows governments to feel safe and emboldened to take the right action. Advocacy from health practitioners allows them to recalibrate the nature of the deal they think they need to strike with their electorates if they are to survive politically, but nevertheless achieve the results we all want.

It might be argued that governments are already under enormous pressure to be bold and that there is little added value in health practitioners setting out their stall. Indeed some governments have already made very bold statements of intent.

Box 5.1
Sweden and Norway

Sweden is to take the biggest energy step of any advanced western economy by trying to wean itself off oil completely by 2020; it is building a new generation of nuclear power stations.

Norway will reduce its emissions of greenhouse gases by 30 per cent by 2020, and be carbon neutral by 2050.

Source: 'Norway carbon neutral by 2050', www.norway.org.uk/policy/news/carbon-neutral.htm; 'Making Sweden an oil free society', www.sweden.gov.se/content/1/c6/06/70/96/7f04f437.pdf

They remain though very largely just that – statements of intent. So whatever the pressure under which governments do already perceive themselves to be, the presure is not yet sufficient to tip them into framing *and implementing* policy likely to lead their country adequately to play its part in global greenhouse gas emission reduction. In the UK for example, many citizens may perceive government policy as being limited to requests, and some incentives, to insulate their homes and drive more efficient cars.

Debating and accepting the need for more government action

Health practitioners in rich countries work in a world shaped by social and political philosophies that value individual choice, rights and freedoms (Hanlon and Carlisle, 2008). So, for example, the freedom to move about by car or plane, without restriction and regardless of the health and ecological consequences, is regarded as right and proper. This has resulted in an emphasis on voluntary behaviour change as a public health response. Yet health practitioners do not flinch from the need to address societal and legal frameworks and structures required to facilitate change, as we can see in tobacco control (which will be discussed later in this chapter) and in pandemic planning.

There is widespread debate about the 'nanny state', which is perceived to interfere with personal liberty and freedom. Some hold the view that 'doing nothing' is the most morally acceptable option in the face of major health issues, as it gives individuals the greatest freedom. However, this does not redress the distribution of power in society that may limit the ability of individuals (particularly vulnerable groups) to act autonomously. Nor does it tackle the determinants of health, such as transport infrastructures, housing, access to low-carbon sources of food etc., which can severely limit people's freedom to live low-carbon, healthy lives.

A fundamental ethical question facing health practitioners is the relationship between the state's authority and the position of individual people and intermediate bodies. At the one end of the spectrum there is a libertarian perspective (which limits involvement in social welfare issues) and at the other is a collectivist point of view (which includes utilitarian or social contract approaches).

The interplay and interaction between individuals, communities and wider populations is central to socio-ecological models of public health. It raises ethical issues about the tension between the individual's rights to freedom and the health of the overall population (that is, in what circumstances an individual's rights can be overridden in the interests of the greater good).

The Nuffield Council on Bioethics (2007) has developed the concept of 'stewardship' by the state to help us address these issues. 'The concept of "stewardship" is intended to convey that liberal states have a duty to look after important needs of people individually and collectively. It emphasises the obligation of states to provide conditions that allow people to be healthy and, in particular, to take measures to reduce health inequalities.'

Core characteristics, proposed by the Nuffield Council, of public health programmes carried out by a stewardship-guided state include:

- Aiming to reduce the risks of ill health by regulations that ensure environmental conditions that sustain good health, such as the provision of clean air and water, safe food and appropriate housing.
- Paying special attention to the health of children and other vulnerable people.
- Promoting health not only by providing information and advice, but also by programmes to help people overcome addictions and

other unhealthy behaviours (and we see our high-carbon lifestyles as 'carbon addiction').

- Aiming to ensure that it is easy for people to lead a healthy life, for example by providing convenient and safe opportunities for walking and cycling.
- Aiming to reduce inequalities that impair health.

The Nuffield Council proposes an 'intervention ladder' (see below) and suggests that substantial restrictions on choice are justified where there is a clear indication that a public health policy will produce the desired effect and has a strong health justification, e.g. prohibiting smoking in enclosed workplaces and public places. It is our belief that the potentially disastrous health impacts of climate change – which threaten our very survival – provide such a justification.

Box 5.2
Nuffield Council on Bioethics –
Public health: Ethical issues, 2007: The intervention ladder

The ladder of possible government actions is as follows:

- Eliminate choice: e.g. prohibiting smoking in enclosed work places and public places, legislating against high CO_2 emitting cars.
- Restrict choice: e.g. industry limits on the fat, salt and sugar content of processed food, or carbon rationing of goods and services.
- Guide choice through disincentives: e.g. tax on cigarettes, congestion charges, taxes on high-carbon goods.
- Guide choice through incentives: e.g. tax breaks on the purchase of bicycles in conjunction with green travel plans.
- Guide choice through changes in policy: e.g. local planning authorities' policies on transport, school catering policies.
- Enable choice: e.g. stop smoking clinics, cycle routes, local food-growing schemes.
- Provide information: e.g. mass-media campaigns.
- Do nothing or monitor the situation: e.g. surveillance of population health.

Nicholas Stern, a former World Bank chief economist, who was commissioned by the UK Government in 2006 to report on the economics of climate change described it as 'the greatest and widest-ranging market failure ever seen' (Stern, 2007). The power of the ethical arguments needs to be put alongside the externalities of climate change, which crucially include destruction of health and an increase in inequalities. We hope you will debate these issues wherever you can, because change has to emerge 'inside out' in a democracy.

The pressures on governments to tackle climate change

To develop an effective strategy for adding to the pressures for bold action by governments we need to understand what those pressures are. There are two main sorts: international and domestic. Both are increasing, especially for the G8, now G20, nations, but are not yet sufficient for us to be confident that the required international action will actually be taken, in time and on a sufficient scale.

International pressures: The United Nations

International pressures include the influence of the United Nations (UN) through individual state membership. This influence is most focused through the UN Framework Convention on Climate Change (UNFCCC), which holds annual major conferences, known as Conferences of the Parties (COPs), themselves based on the work of the Intergovernmental Panel on Climate Change, established by the UN in 1988.

The most concrete output from the UN so far has been the Kyoto Protocol in 1997, implemented in 2005, but giving rise to binding targets only for countries that in total are responsible for about 30 per cent of greenhouse gas emissions (Ministry of Environment, Sweden, 2008). Several nations refused to sign up, notably the US. It is on the replacement of the Kyoto Protocol, which runs out in 2012, that the current series of UNCOPs are engaged. The Bali conference in 2007 produced an important statement of intent to try to forge an international agreement on a global greenhouse gas emissions cap. The Poznan conference in December 2008 was essentially a ground-clearing opportunity in anticipation of the conference in Copenhagen in December 2009. This has been described by many as a 'last chance saloon', if international agreement to a global emission cap is to be achieved *and implemented* in time to reduce the dangerous risks of runaway climate change.

Whilst the contribution of many government delegations to recent conferences demonstrates their determination to achieve this objective, there remains a question mark over the force of such determination when member states return home. Whilst some continue to drag their feet, it is only too easy for others to invoke the 'I will, but only if you will' argument as a basis for inertia.

The recent dramatic deterioration in the global economy has provided even more pretext. There are at least two potent, and international, sources of reinforcement for those states wanting to make progress. Both speak to the heart of the objections to action from countries such as the US (at least until the current presidency). The first comes from the big global corporations, the second – the kernel of this chapter – from the 'health lobby'.

In 2003 global businesses collaborated to form the Climate Group (Climate Group, 2003). Its goal is to help government and business set the world economy on the path to a low-carbon, prosperous future. Just before the Bali UNCOP in December 2007, in an initiative led by the Prince of Wales's UK and European Union Corporate Leaders Groups on Climate Change and the University of Cambridge Programme for Industry, more than 150 chief executives of major British and other corporations signed a communiqué (Bali communiqué, 2007), urging the delegates to be bold, since the alternative was essentially anti-competitive and would harm productivity and growth. In articulating the argument in this way, they were essentially echoing the conclusion of the Stern Report (Stern, 2007) that the costs of failing to take actions to mitigate climate change were several times greater than the costs of mitigation. The health arguments are set out in Chapters 2, 3 and 4 of this book. Their deployment at the Bali UNCOP was on a much more limited scale than that of the Prince of Wales's UK and EU Corporate Leaders Groups on Climate Change. They are international in their application, and it is a core aim of this book to get them deployed more effectively in future.

International pressures: The European Union

The EU has proposed (January 2009) reductions in greenhouse gas emissions of 20 per cent from 1990 levels by 2020, a reduction that is widely believed to be insufficient to prevent runaway climate change. (In 1990, global greenhouse gas emissions were 25 per cent lower than they are now.) The EU looks to be beating a hasty retreat from ambitious emission reduction goals in the belief that the goals will be hugely economically challenging in tough economic times. The EU has also been criticized for failing to provide sufficient funds to help tackle climate change. It has no real strategy to reach the target to which it is rhetorically committed. (The revolt against tough emission reductions targets was led by Germany, Italy and Poland and included all the former communist countries: Hungary, Bulgaria, Estonia, Latvia, Lithuania, Romania and Slovakia. They believe that the cost of additional emission reductions will harm their economies, that is, that energy-intensive industry will be forced to exit Europe and set up in parts of the world where there will be no carbon charge – see www.euractiv.com.)

For member states that have made much of the running in trying to get sign up to a policy of a 20 per cent reduction in emissions by 2020, the feasibility of implementing a strong line domestically is reduced by weak EU decision-making. Potentially, though, the EU represents an enormously important source of pressure on individual member state governments, not least because their own interests are represented as part of a consolidated EU position by the country holding the EU presidency at the time of UNFCOP meetings.

Domestic pressures on governments: The United Kingdom

Within the UK these can be thought of as essentially 'Whitehall-based' and 'citizen-based'. Both types of pressure on government are growing and similar pressures can be found around the world.

Pressure from within

The Whitehall-based pressures include all the structures and processes established by the government itself, reporting to the government or applying pressure on government as part of parliamentary reality. The government department with the lead on climate change issues, the Department for Energy and Climate Change, was created in October 2008. It is the home of the Office of Climate Change, which describes itself as a shared resource across government departments, especially Environment, Food and Rural Affairs (Defra), Business, Enterprise and Regulatory Reform (BERR), Foreign and Commonwealth Office

(FCO), Department for International Development (DFID), Department for Transport (DfT), and Communities and Local Government (Communities).

Defra had previously been the sponsor department for the development and implementation of the government's Sustainable Development Strategy. Significant sums of taxpayers' money were spent on funding highly productive research programmes, for example the Sustainable Technologies Programme, which produced findings incorporated into the UK Sustainable Development Strategy, 'Securing the Future' (Defra, 2005) (see Chapter 3). Its implementation has been faltering and is underfunded.

In addition the Climate Change Act, which passed into law in 2008, has established an independent statutory body, the Committee on Climate Change 'to advise the government on setting and achieving emissions reduction targets'. The act sets legally binding CO_2 emission reduction targets on the government and a system of legally binding five-year 'carbon budgets', set at least 15 years ahead, 'to provide clarity on the UK's pathway towards its key targets' (Defra, 2008). The act has been described as a world first in terms of the statutory obligations it imposes on government.

We wait to see how effective both the act and the Committee turn out to be. The first report of the Committee on Climate Change suggests it intends to exercise its independence. It states that achieving an 80 per cent cut by 2050 is challenging but feasible and is likely to cost between 1 per cent and 2 per cent of the UK's gross domestic product in 2050. Its advice to government on the first carbon budget is, importantly, conditional on reaching a global deal at the UNCOP in Copenhagen in December 2009 and proposes reducing emissions of greenhouse gases by 31 per cent by 2020 below 2005 levels. Very importantly, whilst we are waiting for a deal, the UK should aim to reduce emissions by 21 per cent by 2020 below 2005 levels (Committee on Climate Change, 2008).

A recent example does not imbue confidence in the determination of the government, however. The British Government had made the abolition of fuel poverty among vulnerable households by 2010 legally binding. It has admitted it will not meet the target. This led to Friends of the Earth and Help the Aged applying to take the government to judicial review. This was turned down. The judge's view was that:

> the government had taken up the challenge to eliminate fuel
> poverty by specifying that it would try, so far as reasonably prac-
> ticable, to achieve the targets... In doing so, it imported a statu-
> tory duty to make those efforts. It did not assume a statutory
> duty to achieve the desired results, whatever the cost.
>
> (www.lawreports.co.uk/WLRD/2008/QBD/oct0.5.htm)

This looks like a worrying precedent.

The establishment of the Committee on Climate Change was at least in part
the result of impressive cross-party work by the All Party Parliamentary Climate
Change Group. In establishing an inquiry into the question 'Is a Cross-Party
Consensus on Climate Change Possible – Or Desirable?' they developed the
recommendation that an independent body, analogous to the Bank of England
Monetary Policy Committee, be created and charged with agreeing UK climate
change targets and the possible means for meeting those targets.

The chairman of the All Party Parliamentary Climate Change group, Colin
Challen MP, published in February 2009 a book entitled *The Politics of Climate
Change – too little too late* (Challen, 2009). We hope he is proved wrong.

Pressure on government by citizens

So what of the pressure on government from citizens? There are three sorts.
The first is the campaigning pressure from the environmental lobby, such as
Greenpeace and Friends of the Earth, as well as specific climate change lobbies,
such as the Global Commons Institute and independent think tanks such as
the New Economics Foundation. Their impact has been significant, specifically
in contributing to the Climate Change Act. The campaign for the Climate
Change Act in the UK was the largest public mobilization in recent times.
Almost 130,000 people asked their MP to support the bill (Hale, 2008).

Perhaps of even more significance has been the support of the law courts for
actions that, if related to other causes, would almost certainly have given rise
to successful prosecutions for criminal damage. In September 2008 six activists
admitted trying to shut down Kingsnorth power station in Kent and painting
'Gordon' down the chimney, in a protest at E.ON's plans to build an even bigger
coal-fired station next door. But a jury of nine were persuaded by the activists'
argument, supported in person by James Hansen, the US climate scientist and

director of the National Aeronautics and Space Administration (NASA), that Greenpeace were legally justified because they were trying to prevent climate change causing greater damage to property around the world. In other words climate change activism was legitimated as a just cause. It reminds us of the power of non-violent direct action.

The third source is from the growing number of groups and communities taking local action designed to reduce the size of their own carbon footprint, for example the Transition Town movement, which are described in Chapter 9.

Put together, these examples of civil society expressing its view and taking action amount to a significant shift. This is reflected in the increasingly non-party political consensus across the UK's and other countries' media that radical action is required. Of the three sources, perhaps it is the support of the law courts, the decision by the 'Kingsnorth jury', which suggests that the UK Government is at last at risk of being overtaken by the electorate in respect of boldness of aspirations and concrete actions.

But there is still limited support for legislation such as environmental taxes, with suspicion of how the money will be used and the motive for action. You don't see many campaigners on the streets for personal carbon allowances or road-user charging. So we have a long way to go in influencing public opinion.

To all of the above sources of pressure on governments to act resolutely must now be added the effects of the current global financial and economic crisis. Among its many profound effects, the two most relevant to global action on climate change are addressed in the next section.

The end of poverty and inequalities?

With impoverished populations in the developing world being the first and hardest hit, climate change is very likely to increase the number of preventable deaths. The gaps in health outcomes will get wider. If we really wish to end poverty in our life time, as suggested by Jeffrey Sachs (Sachs, 2005) we will have to ensure that the approach to climate change and inequality is integrated, as we discuss in the following sections.

All 191 UN member states unanimously agreed to the eight Millennium Development Goals by signing the United Nations Millennium Declaration in 2002. In doing so they committed by 2025 to ending the plight of the one sixth of humanity that lives in extreme poverty and struggles daily for survival, and cutting poverty by half by 2015. Sachs also argues strongly for ensuring that all the world's poor, including those in 'moderate' poverty, have a chance to climb the ladder of development. He estimates the cost of meeting the Millennium Development Goals as $135 billion per year in 2006, increasing to $195 billion by 2015. This is between 0.44 and 0.54 per cent of the projected rich world gross national product (GNP) during the decade 2005–2015. This is much less that the 0.7 per cent of GNP already promised as official development assistance (which would be closer to $235 billion at 2003 prices).

These sums should also be set alongside the trillions of dollars found by governments across the world to ease the credit crunch and banking crisis. They should also be compared with the USA' trillion dollar defence budget (Higgs, 2007). In the context of the world's economic problems, the short-term prospects of the rich world spending even 0.5 per cent of GNP on development assistance look diminished.

This opportunity for ending world poverty comes at a time when in the developed world two other phenomena are beginning increasingly to preoccupy politicians. The first is the growing realization that economic growth cannot be seen as an end in itself. More growth not only leads to more and more negative externalities (that is, external impacts on people, communities and the environment), which themselves are obviously destroying the biosphere, but in doing so growth does not even make us happier. On the contrary, as Porritt and others point out (Layard, 2005; Porritt, 2007) the opposite is true (see also the section on mental health in Chapter 4).

The second phenomenon is the growth in social, health and income inequalities worldwide: the gap between rich and poor both globally and within countries. The numbers living in extreme poverty and as a share of the population is rising in Africa (though falling in Asia). The number of people outside China living below $2 per day is reported to have increased from 1,583 million in 1981 to 1,828 million in 1990 and to 2,081 million in 2004 (Pogge, 2008). A third of all human deaths, 18 million annually, are due to poverty-related causes, easily avoidable through better nutrition, safe drinking water, rehydration packs, vaccines, antibiotics and other medicines. At the same time the share of US income of the top 1 per cent of US taxpayers has doubled since 1980.

Table 5.1 Increasing income inequality among countries

Gross national income per capita in nominal US$

Year	Richest countries*	Poorest countries*	Ratio
1980	US$11,840	US$196	60
2000	US$31,522	US$274	115
2005	US$40,730	US$334	122

Notes: *Containing 10 per cent of the world's population. Data derived from Table 1 in the World Bank's World Development Reports for 1982, 2002, and 2007, respectively, and market exchange rates in the relevant years. The ratios among these nominal US$ figures are comparable across years.

Source: reprinted, with permission of the publisher, from Pogge (2008)

The trend and the scale of global inequality is truly staggering. Doubling the wealth of all in the bottom 40 per cent of the population would take only 1.55 per cent of the wealth of the top 1 per cent of the human population. Doubling the wealth of all in the bottom *80* per cent would still take just 15.3 per cent of the wealth of the top 1 per cent.

Within countries, the story is no happier. In China growth has been spectacular, but associated with a great increase in the wealth gap between rich and poor. In the UK your educational attainment, how much you earn and how long you live have become more, not less, a function of your parents' experience over the last 30 years. An Organisation for Economic Co-operation and Development (OECD) report from 2007 surveying all known international studies on mobility in OECD countries, mainly focusing on those born in the 1950s and 1960s, finds that the UK has the lowest change in income between generations of 12 advanced countries (D'Addio, 2007). Worse still, inequality in income has increased at the same time as changes in income from one generation to the next have declined (Blanden et al., 2005).

What's so special about health arguments?

There are three special characteristics of the arguments for radical action particularly, though of course not exclusively, at the disposal of health practitioners:

- The first springs from the powerful point that much of what we should be doing to mitigate climate change globally, nationally, locally and personally, we should be doing anyway for good public health reasons. This is the 'health benefits' argument.
- The second characteristic springs from the *content* of the health-based arguments.
- The third characteristic is the *force* with which they can be delivered to governments – and the electorate.

The health benefits argument

Essentially the argument is that even without the added imperative to mitigate climate change, rich societies are failing adequately to improve, or even protect, their citizens' health, let alone that of the citizens of poorer societies. Taken in the round, our social organization and attitudes and the economy on which they are based, create unhealthy, obesity-causing, inequality-generating, and unsustainable lifestyles. (Readers are referred to Chapter 4 for a detailed description.)

Those things we should be doing to address these health challenges are some of the very same things we should be doing to prevent runaway climate change. The industrialization of agriculture, the unsustainably high, and rapidly increasing, levels of meat consumption promoted through grain subsidies, our tolerance of deaths due to low incomes, cold and road injuries and our lack of global focus on the urgent issues of population stabilization and poverty reduction, are all examples of the behaviour of rich countries likely to make both climate change and global health much worse.

The content of the health arguments

The second important characteristic of the health arguments is the language in which they are couched. It tends to be a language of hope, of better things, of longer lives, quality of life and freedom from disease, as well as of social justice. This is in contrast to the language used in some of the communication on how to stop climate change, which can be about 'giving up', 'rationing' and making do with less.

There are two further key points. The benefits of personal efforts to improve health are likely to accrue personally, often quite quickly. The benefits of personal efforts to prevent climate change are not perceived to benefit individuals in the shorter term at least. People find it hard to make changes sold as benefiting their grandchildren.

Secondly, we have known for some time what we need to do to improve our health, though shamefully in the case of tobacco, worldwide consumption continues to increase (WHO, 2008a). Those things we should change to mitigate climate change have only relatively recently been recognized and in some cases – air travel for example – have increasingly become icons of modern life.

However, it is also true that the language we have developed to combat cigarette consumption is very similar to the language we should be encouraging ourselves and governments to use with respect to climate change reduction: if you stop smoking by age 35, your risk of harm and life expectancy return to normal within a few years and a further benefit is that nobody else suffers the harmful effects of exposure to your smoke. If you drive your car less, take more exercise and eat less meat, you will avoid the effects of obesity and help reduce the effects of climate change. Both sets of changes will help you enjoy your grandchildren and if you reduce your carbon footprint, your grandchildren may have a planet to enjoy (Gill, 2008).

In summary, health-based arguments may be inherently more attractive to people than climate-change-based ones. They may therefore be more persuasive and, if used by politicians, carry less risk of them being tarred with the brush of the 'nanny state'.

The force of health-based arguments

Repeated polls in the UK since 1983 by Ipsos MORI show that the professional most trusted by the public is the doctor (Ipsos Mori, 2007).The effects of well-publicized disasters such as the high mortality rate among children undergoing complex heart surgery at the Bristol Royal Infirmary between 1988 and 1995 and the serial murders of at least 15, and probably many more, patients by their general practitioner, Dr. Harold Shipman during the 1990s have never toppled the medical profession from this position: around 92 per cent of the public believe doctors tell the truth.

Politicians on the other hand, including government ministers, have bumped along the bottom of the list, together with journalists. Only around one in five members of the public believe they tell the truth. A similar position obtains in the USA, where nurses, pharmacists and doctors are regularly in the top five of 21 professions thought by the public to have the highest honesty and ethical standards (American Medical Association, 2005).

Whatever the reasons behind this degree of public trust, it is relevant that health practitioners try to base as much as possible of what they say to the public and to their patients on what the evidence suggests. The prominence of evidence in health and health care systems is exemplified by organizations such as the National Institute for Health and Clinical Excellence in England, the Haute Autorité de la Santé in France and the Agency for Drugs and Technologies in Health in Canada. All have been set up to give clear and authoritative advice on the clinical and cost-effectiveness of interventions.

This prominence of evidence and the reliance on a proper scientific underpinning is something most of us now take for granted, but as the next section suggests, it can on occasions be a two-edged sword.

The other factors contributing to the force of the health messages include:

- The very large number of health practitioners. In the UK alone there are 150,000 doctors and the National Health Service employs over 1.3 million people, as well as all the health practitioners in local government and voluntary and community organizations. The potential power of unanimity, if ever it can be achieved, is obvious.
- The fact that health practitioners are reasonably well organized, for example through their professional associations and colleges, and enjoy access to the national seats of power and influence on a scale as great as any profession.
- The fact that the overwhelming majority of health practitioners are value-driven: they see health protection, poverty reduction and saving the planet not just as technical issues, but fundamentally as issues of social justice.

However, if health practitioners command such trust, base what they do on evidence to such an extent, and have such organized and effective access to power, why for example did it take so long in the UK to enact legislation prohibiting smoking in enclosed workplaces and public places? The answer to this question goes some way to explaining why there is still some difficulty in generating consensus on the scientific evidence relating to climate change. The next section attempts to answer it.

Learning from the past: Overcoming the 'manufacture of uncertainty'

The protection of the public's health often requires decisions to be taken on the precautionary principle: when there is a real risk to health, a decision on whether and how to reduce that risk has to be taken on the best evidence available. This may be less than ideal. It may be incomplete. It may admit of uncertainty. But the more serious the risk associated with inaction, the greater the uncertainty that can be accepted. This is a fundamental principle of public health practice. Unfortunately precisely because risk estimation is often imprecise, and the evidence available may not justify 'certainty' – for example precisely which ingredients in cigarettes cause lung cancer or heart disease – there is an opportunity for those with vested interests to play on this lack of certainty.

This was what happened for more than 40 years: the tobacco industry hired 'scientists' who challenged, distorted and denigrated the growing scientific consensus. This delayed the introduction of evidence-based regulation. Many people died unnecessarily (Michael, 2008).

Arguably it was not until the risks associated with second-hand smoke impinged on citizens' consciousness, particularly non-smoking citizens, by then a clear majority, that governments felt confident in imposing control measures. By this stage the breadth of support had extended from grass-roots advocacy movements, such as BUGA–UP (Billboard Utilising Graffitists against Unhealthy Promotions) in Australia through to the World Health Organization Framework Convention on Tobacco Control.

But even where the science was clearly much better than 'good enough' to justify action, and where the position of health professionals was unanimous,

> **Box 5.3**
> **Uncertainty and action**
>
> As Sir Austin Bradford Hill, a distinguished medical statistician who, with Sir Richard Doll, pioneered the use of the clinical trial and showed the link between smoking and lung cancer, said:
>
> > All scientific work is incomplete – whether it be observational or experimental. All scientific work is liable to be upset or modified by advancing knowledge. That does not confer upon us a freedom to ignore the knowledge we already have, or to postpone action that it appears to demand at a given time... Who knows, asked Robert Browning, but the world may end tonight? True, but on available evidence most of us make ready to commute on the 8:30 next day.
> >
> > (Hill, 1965)

the destructive influence of 'manufactured doubt' delayed proper regulation. There are numerous other examples, including vinyl chloride and asbestos, where the same uncertainty-generating techniques have been used by 'scientists' hired by the industry under threat.

Of more direct relevance to the issue of climate change science is the protracted and still not completely resolved issue of whether and to what extent we should limit our saturated fat intake, if we are to reduce our risk of developing type 2 diabetes and cardiovascular disease. As meat consumption and affluence generally have increased in North America and much of Europe, so too has our intake of saturated fat. Ever since the publication of the National Advisory Committee on Nutrition Education (NACNE) and Committee on Medical Aspects of Food (COMA) reports in the UK (NACNE, 1983; Department of Health, 1984), there has been clear advice to reduce saturated fat intake and by specified amounts. But today less than 4 per cent of adults in Britain have reduced their daily intake to less than 10 per cent of total energy, as recommended (Food Standards Agency, 2004). Why?

There are two main reasons. Firstly there is a significant minority of health professionals, and the public, who remain sceptical. Their arguments often have a plausibility about them that may make them hard to counter, at least in simple language. Why for example are heart disease death rates in France lower than in England, when we know they eat large quantities of butter,

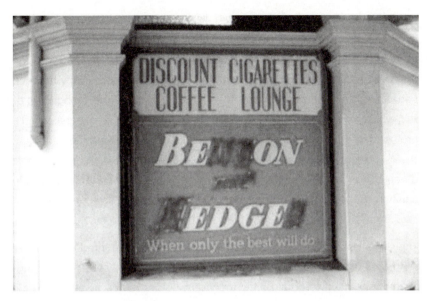

Figure 5.1 Example of BUGA–UP activity: Grass-roots advocacy

Source: found at www.bugaup.org/gallery.htm (permission not sought)

cream and meat in France? Secondly government policy is inconsistent. On the one hand we are advised to eat less saturated fat. On the other there are large subsidies on both sides of the Atlantic for the production of animal feed and this directly encourages yet more meat consumption.

If there is a vested interest, if the message involves doing less of something, particularly something we like, or which confers status, and if the science underpinning the message uses words such as 'probable' rather than 'certain', initiating behaviour change at individual or political level tends to be hampered by the gainsayers, the opponents.

The strategy of the global warming deniers is painfully reminiscent of that used by the tobacco industry. For example, as recently as November 2006 the US Deputy Solicitor General Gregory C. Garre, acting for the government against 12 states and 13 public interest groups in the Supreme Court, invoked scientific uncertainty as one of the reasons the Environmental Protection Agency should not be compelled to treat the greenhouse gas carbon dioxide as a pollutant (Michael, 2006), despite all the scientific evidence reviewed in Chapter 1.

Behind the political power of the evidence on the health impacts of second-hand smoke was the fear non-smokers began legitimately to feel that they would be harmed, even lose their lives. It was fear that, lay behind the legitimacy and the effectiveness of the UK Government's actions in the mid-1980s to try to prevent AIDS. 'Don't Die of Ignorance', a public awareness campaign that involved TV adverts and leaflets through every letter box, clearly changed behaviour. Although the target of the campaign was HIV (new diagnoses of HIV, which were over 3,000 in 1985, dropped by a third in three years), it had a profound effect on all sexually transmitted infections: following the campaign, the number of diagnoses of gonorrhoea in England and Wales for example dropped from around 50,000 in 1985 to just 18,000 in 1988 (BBC, 2009). In addition to the campaign, large sums of money were found for research, for care (there was no effective treatment then) and for surveillance.

This surveillance involved collecting data from individuals not just on their HIV status, but on the type of behaviour that might alter it, whether sexual or drug-related. The need to obtain patient consent before testing assumed a huge new prominence. The public, though, seemed to understand that we knew little about the disease, were worried they could contract it and apparently accepted that surveillance was fundamental to our knowing how to limit the damage of the epidemic.

So even though there was huge uncertainty and lack of knowledge about the nature of the threat of HIV/AIDS, the gainsayers had little hope of making their case heard. For in addition to the fear, there was a clear liberal scientific consensus that developed on the importance of 'safe sex'. With strong urging from the Chief Medical Officer and very senior civil servants the British Government had little compunction in taking bold action.

Our challenge now is to urge governments to respond in the same bold way in dealing with the global threats of climate change, persisting poverty and increasing inequalities. We know many of the ingredients of the equivalent of safe sex in reducing greenhouse gas emissions. We have no cure for runaway climate change. The public is afraid, but not at quite such a personal level as with HIV. The climate change deniers are still out there, but the Intergovernmental Panel on Climate Change 4th report (see Chapter 1) has done much to establish consensus. And the US administration that did so much to foster the uncertainty is no longer in power.

Implications for health practitioners

This chapter has so far argued that:

- Health practitioners have a distinctive contribution to make to tackling climate change.
- Many of the things we all need to do across the world to stop climate change we should be doing anyway, to protect and promote public health.

By *not* taking action, and being seen not to take action by the public, we will be transmitting a powerful and unintended message. When doctors smoked in front of their patients, it signified that in the minds of the profession the risks of smoking to health were small. If doctors and other health practitioners do not demonstrate personally the importance of our individual and collective carbon footprints to health, a similar misapprehension will be perpetuated. We have to show leadership on this issue, just as we did for many of the scourges of the past.

Our record in hastening the end of many of these scourges has been impressive. The sanitary revolution in the 19th century, and the control of smallpox in the 20th century stand out. But in other areas the threat to health has not given rise to an effective assault by health practitioners – for example, the persisting and increasing scar of inequalities and the compelling threat to health of nuclear war. Our professional voice has been less forceful, our personal commitment equivocal and our advocacy half-hearted.

So, at least until now, it is with climate change. To enable us to exert the influence that we are capable of, we must have the moral and intellectual courage to:

- illustrate the clear links;
- articulate the major benefits of appropriate action;
- lead personal life styles that are climate-friendly;
- sharpen our advocacy.

What does this mean in practice?

How can we mobilize ourselves?

To harness the very considerable potential of health practitioners to make a huge difference, we propose a five pronged approach:

1   Health practitioners need to INFORM – to be clear to the public, to patients and to politicians about the risks of doing nothing and about the benefits to both individual and global health of effective action. 'Deniers' need to be tackled head on. We must use the evidence summarized in Part I of this book to generate consensus and reduce the opportunities for the manufacture of uncertainty.

2   Health practitioners need to AFFIRM – to give a lead through personal actions and exert influence on the organizations within which they work. The power of leadership by example is not to be underestimated. It is about living our values for real.

3   Health practitioners need to ADVOCATE, for the development and especially the implementation of a health-promoting global framework, grounded in social justice. Advocacy must be directed at those best placed to influence the political process, particularly elected officials. It must be based on the tried and tested elements known to be effective: being specific, brief, personal, timely, confident and, crucially, factual. Accuracy is vital.

4   We need to INNOVATE, by using imaginative ways to amplify the voice of health practitioners. For example, some believe that the speed with which a relatively small number of demonstrators (initially perhaps as few as 2500) brought the country, and the government, to their knees in a matter of days in the UK fuel dispute in 2000 was in large measure due to the use of the mobile phone.

5   Health practitioners need to disseminate the message, its significance to us all and its urgency, by using all our extensive networks. We need to seek new ways of using these networks to coordinate activities and link with the many others who share the commitment to tackle climate change.

The need for urgent action is clear. We know what interventions are needed. We must above all not only agree but *implement* a global framework that constrains global carbon emissions but does not constrain the development of those countries where many struggle to survive, particularly in sub-Saharan Africa. The framework must therefore require both a major reduction in carbon emissions from the rich world and enable a rise in emissions for the poor world, which is very small in global terms and in any case temporary, but crucial for their development.

Solutions must be integrated, preventive and universal

As climate change and poverty are global issues, solutions promoted by the global framework must be:

- integrated, so ensuring that tackling one problem does not exacerbate another;
- preventive, so minimizing the possibility of the solutions giving rise to new problems;
- universal, which can only be achieved when the global community brokers a deal that is supported by all the nations.

The only realistic forum for effecting such a framework at present is the UN, through the UNFCCC (United Nations Framework Convention on Climate Change). This international forum meets most years at the Conference of the Parties (COP) and is the organization that hammered out the Kyoto Protocol in 1997, the only international agreement reached so far. The next COP conference in Copenhagen in December 2009 (COP 15) is, many think, our last chance to gain agreement to cap global emissions. It is towards the end of our 'golden hour', the time available following acute injury to increase the victim's chances of survival by aggressive treatment.

Each country has political and technical representation at these conferences. Many non-governmental organizations (NGOs) are involved. Part of our strategy must be to support their initiatives, but it is the governments' delegates and their technical advisors who carry most clout. Our advocacy must be directed at those politicians closely involved in the moulding of the Copenhagen resolutions and their implementation thereafter.

143

Influencing the political process

The ingredients of the framework

Politicians, even when well disposed towards the issues of climate change, poverty and inequality, will not listen to us unless we have a scientifically credible story to tell, a story supported by good research and articulated clearly by large numbers of our organizations and individual health professionals. To engage their attention in the overcrowded world of climate change politics, we must also be able to set out the ingredients of the healing framework we believe to be necessary.

We believe any framework must have the following three ingredients:

1   First and foremost, a scientifically assessed and globally binding commitment to cap and reduce carbon emissions to avoid atmospheric concentrations greater than 350–450 parts per million, to give ourselves a high probability of limiting average global temperature rises to 2–2.4°C.

2   A mechanism for ensuring that resources are transferred to those countries where both living standards and fossil fuel use have been low. These resources include support to enable population stabilization, which is essential to the future health of the planet (see Chapter 4).

3   An approach to development that, by giving people the capability of making low-carbon choices, minimizes greenhouse gas emissions.

The 'fair shares' Contraction and Convergence framework articulated by the Global Commons Institute (www.GCI.org.uk), is founded on these three principles and is the most feasible present option (see Chapter 4 for more information). If other frameworks emerge that have these three ingredients, we must support them.

Demonstrating health professional support

We must also be able to show the politicians the extent of health professional support for our position. There is plenty of exhortation, notably from the Director General of the World Health Organization, Dr Margaret Chan, who said in December 2007 that climate change was 'the defining issue for public health during this century'. She went on to say:

> The health sector must add its voice – loud and clear – to the growing concern ... we must fight to place health issues at the centre of the climate agenda. We have compelling reasons for doing so. Climate change will affect, in profoundly adverse ways, some of the most fundamental determinants of health: food, air, water. (Chan, 2007)

World Health Day in 2008 was dedicated to protecting health from climate change and the 61st World Health Assembly in May 2008 adopted a resolution urging member states to take decisive action to address health impacts from climate change.

Relevant information has been collated in this book and in the sources to which it refers. At the time of writing, a study is underway to pull together a concise statement of the health and economic benefits of the actions we propose, as well as the consequences of inaction. This should build on the Stern report (Stern, 2007).

Now that we are clear about what it is we are asking for, and armed with the evidence base we have collated in this book, how do we garner support for our proposals from organizations and individuals across the world?

For example in the UK, there are a number of health-based networks including the Sustainable Development Commission; the Health and Sustainable Development Network; Medact; the student organization Medsin and the Green Alliance. Networks in other countries include Physicians for Social Responsibility in the USA; International Society of Doctors for the Environment (ISDE), based in Switzerland; the Health and Environment Alliance, based in Brussels and Health Care Without Harm, a global coalition, working in more than 50 countries (see the resources section at end of book).

In the UK, the NHS Sustainable Development Unit, established in 2008, develops organizations, people, tools, policy and research to help the National Health Service in Britain fulfil its potential as a leading sustainable and low-carbon organization. The NHS Carbon Reduction Strategy, Saving Carbon, Improving Health (NHS SDU, 2008) is described in Chapters 1 and 11. The Carbon Trust works directly with many NHS organizations to provide practical information and support on carbon reduction.

Increasing numbers of health professionals and health organizations have joined the Climate and Health Council. The Council is a charitable organization overseen by a board of prominent health professionals and students, chosen for their individual commitment as well as for their organizational links. It seeks to articulate and coordinate the activities of health professionals in combating climate change. The council has developed a declaration setting out:

- the health perils we face if we do not act in an integrated way on climate change, poverty and inequality;
- the benefits of action;
- the need for a 'fair shares' health-promoting framework.

Membership of the council is open to any health professional, student or manager, simply by supporting the Declaration on the website (www.climate-andhealth.org).The council has asked as many health professionals as possible to sign a pledge (see below).

The council is feeding this demonstration of the breadth and depth of support from health professionals into the negotiations before, during and after the United Nations Conference of the Parties in Copenhagen in November 2009.

Box 5.4

Climate and Health Council Pledge

To protect health through active engagement to limit the causes of human-caused climate change and to advocate:

- the establishment of a global, systematic and consistent approach, led and implemented by governments NOW, based on an agreed global framework;
- the redistribution of resources.

We believe this model could, with appropriate modification, be replicated throughout the world, forming a coalition of councils or associations linked at least through the internet and deploying the power, for example, of web-based tools such as Facebook and Myspace.

Influencing the politicians

Clarity about our ambition, a strong body of documentary evidence and the fact of widespread support, together form a sound base from which to influence the political process. In England the Climate and Health Council Board includes several distinguished leaders of the medical profession, such as the President of the Royal College of Physicians, editors of the *British Medical Journal* and *The Lancet* and medical students.

Students are of particular importance, not only because they represent the generation that has most to gain and lose, and whose voice is not usually given enough prominence, but also for their energy and their insights into new ways of networking. The composition of the board thus gives the council access to the corridors of power through several routes.

Box 5.5
Guidance from nature: Fractals

We can be guided by examples from nature. Fractals, structures that appear similar at all levels of magnification, are an essential ingredient of the make up of the natural world. Good examples are cauliflowers, snowflakes and mountain ranges.

Our actions should likewise embed consistency across size and range, from the personal through the local and regional to the global.

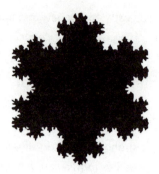

Figure 5.2 A Koch snowflake, constructed from equilateral triangles

The approach outlined in this section reflects our UK base. The themes and principles are applicable elsewhere. Our aim should be to exert pressure on an international and coordinated basis.

In the UK, approaching our elected officials – councillors, members of UK and European parliaments – is an easy first step. We need to press for proper implementation of the UK Climate Change Act and for a negotiating position to be adopted by both the UK and the EU at the Copenhagen Conference of the Parties on Climate Change – and subsequent negotiations – that reflects the framework above.

A good first step in the UK is to meet your local member of parliament, or in other countries your elected official. Tell him or her that health practitioners are taking climate change seriously and describe the health impacts (Chapter 2) and the health benefits (Chapter 4). Say that the NHS is taking action (Chapter 11) but that we urgently need stronger government support.

Other routes include those involving officials – civil servants – in government departments. In the UK the Department of Health (DH) is not the lead government department on climate change negotiations, but it nevertheless has an important role. It represents the United Kingdom in the World Health Organization and has cross-Whitehall responsibilities. We must therefore persuade the DH to take a lead in bringing to the fore the health dimensions of climate change and to emphasize the need for the Kyoto Treaty to be replaced by an agreement rooted in considerations of global health. It needs to be seen to be actively supporting the efforts of the UK Sustainable Development Commission, the NHS Sustainable Development Unit and other active bodies.

In concert with our approach to the DH, we must talk to those in the Department of Energy and Climate Change and the Foreign and Commonwealth Office who are more directly concerned with the Copenhagen negotiations.

Outside the UK, we should be attracting the attention of other important actors, such as:

- Gro Brundtland, one of the three UN special envoys on climate change and a former Director General of the WHO.
- Yvo de Boer, the Dutch executive director of the UNFCCC and so the United Nations 'climate chief'.
- Achim Steiner, the executive director of the UN environment programme with a special interest in sustainable development, and an appreciation that healthy societies and sustainable societies share the same social, environmental and economic structure.

Synergy with other professions and groups

Health practitioners are only one of many groups pressing for change. Our voice will be greatly amplified if we act with other professionals, such as architects, engineers and teachers. For instance The Royal Institute of British Architects (RIBA) advocates for a fair shares agreement and is a willing partner in cooperative advocacy (RIBA, 2009).

The political clout of the business community is arguably hugely greater than that of health practitioners. We need to collaborate with the business community to develop arguments that link politically attractive, because immediate, economic gains with long-term social and environmental good. Investment in renewable energy and the green economy are good examples. Investment in low-carbon industries and jobs is at the heart of the fiscal stimulus package being negotiated by US President Obama (see Larry Elliot and Andrew Simms (2008) who plot this way forward in the UK).

Towards a global social movement

The more countries in which this sort of approach to advocacy can be replicated the better. All should ultimately be involved, but there may be mileage in collaborative advocacy with those countries that have shown support for a global framework incorporating the three ingredients that we advocate: South

Africa, Mexico, Brazil, Switzerland and Norway. No global deal is going to be possible, however, without leadership from China, the EU, India and the USA. Pressure by health professionals from these countries on their representatives in international agencies is particularly important. Extensive international medical and medical student networks can be activated by committed supporters within them. Health professionals who are concerned about the issues discussed in this chapter can also be identified within international agencies such as the World Health Organization.

A sustained campaign

Even if a global agreement to a carbon cap and a continual reduction in global emissions is reached at the UNFCCC in Copenhagen, political leaders will need all the support they can get to ensure the implementation of the agreed policy. Indeed one political analysis is that such an agreement might well produce an electoral backlash, as implementation of the necessary measures may be felt as real constraints on individual lifestyles, particularly in developed economies. To attain this increased support we should develop several further initiatives.

Engaging more and more health practitioners

We must continue to recruit an ever increasing number of health practitioners, particularly colleagues in the poorer parts of the world. Many of the professional associations based in rich northern countries have extensive membership all over the world. We must redouble our efforts to engage this membership, encouraging them to act as catalysts for the formation of organizations similar to the UK Climate and Health Council.

Communicating the health benefits

Transmitting our information about the enormous health benefits that could accrue from tackling climate change, and our passion for action, will be at the heart of our networking campaign. Health practitioners must look to the success of the Obama campaign, which was built on Howard Dean's campaign for the democratic presidential nomination in 2004 (Dean's Campaign, 2009), for ideas on viral networking.

Supporting non-violent direct action campaigns

Given the mismatch between political inertia and the gravity of our predicament, an increase is anticipated in the number of non-violent direct actions directed against installations that are profligate in emitting CO_2. Health professionals should support these campaigns by making the health case against, for instance, airport expansion and coal-powered electricity generation without carbon capture and storage.

We can argue that the perpetrators of non-violent direct action do so in the public health interest and therefore are not committing a criminal offence, but are on the contrary acting out of necessity. As mentioned earlier, we have the example of Kingsnorth where the protestors were acquitted by a jury on the grounds that their actions were for the greater good. What greater good is there than the health of humanity?

Health practitioners can also support the Global Day of Action Campaign, (www.globalclimatecampaign.org). This campaign coordinates annual days of demonstration and action around the world, at the time of the annual UN Framework Convention on Climate Conference negotiations.

Advocacy to reduce consumption of pharmaceuticals

The largest component of the health service carbon footprint in the UK is generated from the life cycle of pharmaceuticals (NHS SDU, 2008 and see Chapter 1), and it is likely that this is the case throughout the rich world. There is a wide variation in consumption of drugs, with people in Germany and France taking many more drugs than in the UK, indicating that the overall consumption of drugs is culturally determined. In view of the high carbon cost of drugs, we must change this culture.

Preventive measures such as eating less meat and exercising more will reduce our need for some drugs, but the effect of any such reduction may well be overtaken by the introduction of new, particularly anti-cancer, drugs. It is estimated that up to 40 per cent of drugs given for chronic conditions in western societies are never taken (Sabaté, 2003). Many drugs, particularly antibiotics and antidepressants, are given inappropriately (Otters et al, 2004) and even when given appropriately there may be low-carbon alternatives, such as talking and walking therapy for mild and moderate depression (Mental Health

Foundation, 2005; Kirsch et al, 2008) and pelargonium tablets for viral afflictions (Lizogub et al, 2007).

Attempts to reduce drug consumption based on these arguments will lead to a backlash from the pharmaceutical companies. They themselves will be under significant pressure to demonstrate their own social and environmental responsibility by developing new low-carbon approaches to drug development, manufacture and distribution.

'Transition Towns' as healthy towns

As described in Chapter 9, health practitioners should link with our colleagues in the 'Transition Town' movement and seek to create a transition health facilities movement, which may stimulate more effective action on redesigning health care.

Renewable energy: Health benefits

The direct health benefits of renewable energy are considerable, particularly in reducing indoor smoke pollution in poor countries (Markandya and Wilkinson, 2007). Health professionals should push for the generation of renewables as a preventive measure.

Engaging with the public

In many countries a large proportion of the population visit a health facility at least once a year and health professionals should use the opportunity of these contacts to engage the wider public. At present primary care facilities in the UK are full of posters and pamphlets about contraception, housing benefits or the dangers of tobacco. We must develop and display an array of materials setting out the health *and* environmental gains associated with, for instance, eating less meat and walking and bicycling rather than driving (see Chapter 4).

Health practitioners should encourage individuals to measure and reduce their personal carbon emissions and link this to the health benefits that are likely to accrue. This is an excellent way of showing individual leadership.

Conclusion: From campaigning to sustained social movement

All the initiatives suggested in this chapter have two complementary objectives:

- The first is to increase the public understanding of the inextricable links between mitigating climate change and protecting global health.
- The second is to make it riskier for politicians to do nothing than for them to be radical on both fronts: health and global warning, both in what they say and in what they do.

These objectives will be best met if health practitioners, individually and collectively, align themselves with all the many other coalitions, organizations and institutions advocating action. In other words health practitioners must play their part in the establishment of a social movement that makes it possible, if not easy, for politicians to do what they have to do, if the planet and humanity are to survive and flourish.

To enable the transition from effective campaigning to sustained social movement, we may well need to redirect our efforts to new groups of politicians and to form new networks. Whatever we do, we must never forget that the opportunity for intervention, the planet's golden hour, is coming perilously close to its end.

Action points

1   Reflect on your own experience of networking and campaigning to achieve changes in health policy or practice. What has been successful and what methods and approaches have been most valuable?
2   Consider your own views on the role of the state or government in achieving a substantial reduction in greenhouse gas emissions – we need to achieve at least a 40 per cent reduction in the next 20 years.
3   How would *you* summarize what is so special and persuasive about the health arguments in influencing public opinion on climate change?

4   How can you personally, perhaps with colleagues, get involved in lobbying for a successful outcome/implementation of the agreement reached at the United Nations in Copenhagen in December 2009?

5   Which politicians could you influence locally, and how?

6   What professional groups, networks or environmental groups do you belong to? Could you get more involved in urging any of them to add their weight to the climate change lobby? Are there other groups you could join?

7   Who can you link up with as a partner in your advocacy to give you confidence?

8   Could you get involved with the Annual Global Day of Action Campaign?

9   Are you in a position to help in any way to reduce the consumption of pharmaceuticals (the largest element of the British National Health Service's carbon footprint?)

10 Are there any specific non-violent direct action campaigns concerning climate change that you might consider getting involved with?

References

American Medical Association (2005) 'Which Professionals does the Public Trust the Most, and the Least?', available at www.ama-assn.org/amednews/2005/01/03/prca0103.htm (accessed 1 March 2009)

Ashton Hayes (2008) available at www.goingcarbonneutral.co.uk (accessed 1 March 2009)

Bali communiqué (2007) available at www.balicommunique.com (accessed 1 March 2009)

BBC (2009) available at http://news.bbc.co.uk/1/hi/programmes/panorama/4348096.stm (accessed 7 February 2009)

Blanden, J., Gregg, P. and Machin, S. (2005) 'Intergenerational Mobility in Europe and North America', report supported by the Sutton Trust, Centre for Economic Performance, London, available at www.suttontrust.com/reports/IntergenerationalMobility.pdf (accessed 1 March 2009)

Challen, C. (2009) The Politics of Climate Change: too little too late, Picnic Publishing, Hove, UK

Chan, M. (2007) 'Climate Change and Health: Preparing for Unprecedented Challenges', available at www.who.int/dg/speeches/2007/20071211_maryland/en/print.html (accessed 1 February 2009)

Climate Group (2003) available at www.theclimategroup.org/ (accessed 1 March 2009)

Committee on Climate Change (2008) 'Building a Low-Carbon Economy – The UK's Contribution to Tackling Climate Change', available at www.theccc.org.uk/reports (accessed 1 February 2009)

D'Addio, A. (2007) 'Intergenerational transmission of disadvantage – mobility or immobility across generations?', a review of the evidence for OECD countries, OECD, Paris

Dean's Campaign (2009) available at www.wired.com/wired/archive/12.01/dean.html (accessed 7 February 2009)

Defra (2005) 'Securing the Future. The UK Government Sustainable Development Strategy', HMSO, London

Defra (2008) available at www.defra.gov.uk (accessed 1 March 2009)

Department of Health (1984) 'Diet and Cardiovascular Disease – Report of the Panel on Diet in Relation to Cardiovascular Disease of the Committee on Medical Aspects of Food Policy', Report on Health and Social Subjects 28, HMSO, London

Elliot, L. and Simms, A. (eds) (2008) *Green New Deal: Joined-up Policies to Solve the Triple Crunch of the Credit Crisis, Climate Change and High Oil Prices*, New Economics Foundation, London

Food Standards Agency (2004) 'The National Diet & Nutrition Survey: adults aged 19 to 64 years', HMSO, London

Gill M. (2008) 'Why should doctors be interested in climate change?', *British Medical Journal*, vol 306, p1506

Hale, S. (2008) *The New Politics of Climate Change: Why We Are Failing and How We Will Succeed,* Green Alliance, London

Hanlon, P. and Carlisle, S. (2008) 'Do we face a third revolution in human history? If so, how will public health respond?', *Journal of Public Health*, vol 30, no 4, pp355–361

Higgs, R. (2007) 'The Trillion-dollar Defense Budget is Already Here', available at www.independent.org/newsroom/article.asp?id=1941 (accessed 1 March 2009)

Hill, A.B. (1965) 'The environment and disease: Association or causation?' *Proceedings of the Royal Society of Medicine*, vol 58, pp295–300

IPCC (2007) 'Climate Change 2007: Synthesis Report', Contribution of Working Groups I, II and III to the Fourth Assessment, Pachauri, R.K and Reisinger, A. (eds) IPCC, Geneva, Switzerland

Ipsos Mori (2007) 'Trust in Professions', available at www.ipsos-mori.com/content/polls-07/trust-in-professions-2007.ashx

Kirsch, I., Deacon, B.J., Huedo-Medina, T.B., Scoboria, A., Moore, T.J. and Johnson, B.J. (2008) 'Initial severity and antidepressant benefits: a meta-analysis of data submitted to the Food and Drug Administration', *PLoS Medicine (Public Library of Science)*, vol 5, no 2, e45

Layard. R, (2005) *Happiness*, Allen Lane, London

Lizogub, V.G., Riley, D.S. and Heger, M. (2007) 'Efficacy of a *Pelargonium sidoides* preparation in patients with the common cold: a randomized, double blind, placebo-controlled clinical trial', *Explore (NY)*, vol 3, pp573–584

Markandya, A. and Willkinson, P. (2007) 'Electricity generation and health', *The Lancet, Energy and Health*, September, pp19–30

Mental Health Foundation (2005) *Exercise Therapy and the Treatment of Mild to Moderate Depression in Primary Care*, Mental Health Foundation, London

Michael, D. (2006) 'Let's Debate the Science – Taking the Tobacco Road to the Supreme Court', available at http://thepumphandle.wordpress.com/2006/12/01/lets-debate-the-science-taking-the-tobacco-road-to-the-supreme-court (accessed 1 March 2009)

Michael, D. (2008) *Doubt is their Product. How Industry's Assault on Science Threatens your Health*, Oxford University Press, Oxford

Ministry of Environment, Sweden (2008) 'The Path Towards a New International Agreement on the Earth's Climate', available at www.regeringen.se/content/1/c6/10/33/83/27418bc4.pdf (accessed 1 March 2009)

NACNE (1983) 'A discussion paper on proposals for nutritional guidelines for health education in Britain', National Advisory Committee on Nutrition Education, Health Education Council, London

NHS SDU (2008) *NHS England Carbon Emissions: carbon footprint study*, Sustainable Development Unit, Sustainable Development Commission and Stockholm Environment Institute, Sustainable Development Unit, London.

Nuffield Council on Bioethics (2007) *Public Health: ethical issues*, Nuffield Council on Bioethics, London

Otters, H.B.M, van der Wouden, J.C., Schellevis, F.G., van Suijlekom-Smit, L.W.A. and Koes, B.W. (2004) 'Trends in prescribing antibiotics for children in Dutch general practice', *Journal of Antimicrobial Chemotherapy*, vol 53, pp361–366

Pogge, T. (2008) 'Growth and inequality: understanding recent trends and political choices', *Dissent Magazine*, available at http://dissentmagazine.org/article/?article=990 (accessed 1 March 2009)

Porritt, J. (2007) *Capitalism as if the World Matters*, 2nd edition, Earthscan, London

RIBA 2009, RIBA Policy, available at www.architecture.com/Files/RIBAHoldings/PolicyAndInternationalRelations/Policy/Environment/ClimateChangePolicy.pdf (accessed 7 February 2009)

Sabaté, E. (ed) (2003) *Adherence to Long Term Therapies: evidence For action*, World Health Organization, Geneva

Sachs, J. (2005) *The End of Poverty: how we can make it happen in our lifetime*, Penguin Books, London

Stern, N. (2007) *The Economics of Climate Change: the stern review*, Cambridge University Press, Cambridge

WHO (2008a) 'WHO Report on the Global Tobacco Epidemic, 2008: The MPower Package', World Health Organization, Geneva

WHO (2008b) 'Closing the gap in a generation: health equity through action on the social determinants of health', Commission on Social Determinants of Health, originally in Pogge, T. (2008)

6

How to Help to Plan a Healthy, Sustainable, Low-carbon Community

Hugh Barton, Marcus Grant
and Philip Insall

Development can literally make communities sick ...
almost every planning decision or policy has a potential effect
on human health.

National Health Service Healthy Urban Development Unit (England)

Summary

If health practitioners can get involved with the strategic planning systems and processes led by local government in their local areas, they can help to ensure that health is central to the design of their local communities. This may sound arid and boring, but it really is very important to creating healthy, sustainable, low-carbon communities! The impacts of climate instability, obesity and other health challenges should be the focus for health practitioner interaction with the planning process. The aim should be to get health and climate change objectives into the key documents, the frameworks and plans, from the outset. If the original objectives are right then the chance of a good outcome for health and climate change is hugely increased. To make the most impact, it is important to get hold of as much detail as possible and meet with the planning officers. It is also vital to reach, and convince, the movers and shakers, such as politicians and chief officers.

Specifically, promoting active travel is hugely important both to avoid runaway climate change and to promote health. Transport should not be thought of as 'mobility' – that is, people in vehicles able to move freely – but 'accessibility', that is, people able to get to the places they want to go. It is not just a matter of an efficient and safe walking, cycling and public transport system. Accessibility demands that we localize as much as possible, making walking and cycling routes shorter and quicker. In future we would no longer need to make so many and such long trips. People tend to overestimate cost and travel time for public transport and underestimate these for their car. Through a combination of individual support for personal travel planning and improvements to the built environment to make walking and cycling and use of public transport easier, there is huge potential for increasing healthy, low-carbon travel. Involvement in planning systems is essential to achieving this outcome.

Be a champion for healthy, sustainable communities in the planning process!

Key terms

Planning: A generic term often used as shorthand for town and country planning or spatial planning.

Town and country planning: The planning of the physical fabric – buildings, spaces, streets, infrastructure, landscape – of urban and rural areas in order to achieve social, economic and environmental goals.

Spatial planning: The term coined in the United Kingdom 2004 Planning Act for town and country planning: implying (in the UK) a holistic approach, with all the agencies collaborating in making decisions about development.

Development: Building, infrastructure and landscape projects that alter the built environment.

Built environment: The whole human-made environment of cities, towns and villages, including landscape features and spaces as well as buildings.

What does a healthy, sustainable, low-carbon community look like?

To set the scene, here are some elements of the communities we are creating through the processes described in this chapter: sustainable, healthy and low-carbon. We are sure you will be able to add to this list. Perhaps the key words are 'local', 'resilient' and 'self-reliant'.

- Communities will be strong, resilient, able to withstand shocks and respond to rapid change, and therefore mutually supportive and integrated.
- Everything we need to live a fulfilling life will be as local as possible.
- All our basic needs will be met: clean air, fresh water, food, housing, income and safety, which will involve some sharing of resources.
- Housing will be well designed and appropriately located; no noise pollution; neighbourhoods will feel safe and secure.
- We will spend much less of our time travelling. The places we need to get to (offices, shops, schools, primary health care, parks etc.) will

be accessible on foot, by bicycle or by public transport. They will be at the appropriate scale to match our needs. As services become more local and journeys shorter, access for people with various forms of restriction to their mobility will also improve. Cars will only be used when no other option is possible.

- Work-related travel will be massively reduced through the wide availability of high-quality video conferencing.
- Household and workplace energy consumption will be dramatically lower, through a combination of retro fitting buildings with insulation and energy-saving technology, and local energy generation.
- As much food as possible will be grown and sourced locally, to improve food quality, provide maximum food security and reduce carbon; gardens will be shared to grow fruit, salads, vegetables and herbs as well as flowers.
- Markets and investment for as many other goods as possible will also be local.
- There will be as many trees, as much green space and nectar-rich planting as can be squeezed in to every corner.
- A wide variety of social and cultural opportunities will be available locally.
- Our health, well-being and quality of life will be greatly improved.

Spatial planning for sustainable development

Given the plethora of terms in current usage to describe planning – town and country, urban, land use, to name but a few – this chapter chooses 'spatial planning', which, as noted above, has been adopted by the United Kingdom (UK) Government. It implies something much broader and deeper than the bureaucratic process of obtaining planning permission. Essentially it is about planning for the future of human settlements (from farmsteads to conurbations). It includes all the facets of settlement, even where responsibility is not traditionally seen as the remit of the local authority planning department: transport, housing, economic development, regeneration, open space and so on.

The prime purpose of planning – as seen in the UK and the European Union – is 'sustainable development'. The accepted United Nations definition is from the Brundtland Report: 'development which meets the needs of the present without compromising the ability of future generations to meet their needs' (World Commission on Environment and Development, 1987). The principle of sustainable development is one to which anyone trying to influence planning decisions can appeal (for more information, see Chapter 3). It is people-centred and thus accords with a health and well-being perspective; and climate change is the biggest driver for the adoption of sustainable development as the goal of planning. This is made quite explicit in a key official UK document: Planning Policy Statement No.1 (PPS1), which is well worth reading – it is not too long (see Office of the Deputy Prime Minister, 2005) and it sets out the purpose and scope of spatial planning.

Of course, we have not always held this broad and deep view of planning in the UK. In the 1980s the view was that planning existed to facilitate economic development and protect what is best in the environment. Health, social justice and quality of life were all excluded. We still live with the aftermath of that belief. Some very influential bodies – in particular the Treasury – still hold on to something similar. Planning authorities therefore often find themselves in a double bind: told by the government that their job is the creation of a healthy, sustainable environment; assessed by government (and, thereby funded) on the basis of purely instrumental criteria – how fast are plans prepared and development control decisions made? The job is not an easy one!

Later sections of this chapter will look in some detail at the British planning system, the main official bodies responsible and the mechanisms that express and implement policy. But it is worth making a much more general point first: 'planning' is just part of the overall 'development process'. To understand what is meant by that term consider how development happens – for example, how does a new housing estate or supermarket get constructed? There is a whole sequence of different interests involved; the landowner, a potential developer (house builder or retailer), a bank or other financial body willing to lend the capital, professionals – planners, architects, engineers, ecologists etc. – advising the developer, construction firms and regulatory bodies (like the Environmental Agency). The local authority, coming into this process, may speak with forked tongue – the policy planners (responsible for the long-term forward plan), the transport engineers (sometimes at the county level – a different authority altogether), the affordable housing professionals, the treasurers (responsible for the public purse) – all have different priorities. The councillors, who have the final say, may also have their own political interests, which cut across all the others.

The point is that plans are only as good as the development decisions that are supposed to implement them. However, plans have to be practicable, working to *mould* market and institutional forces, not block them. Health practitioners getting involved in this process, as we hope you will, may find allies in unlikely quarters. For example the planning consultants advising their developer clients may be grateful for support in highlighting health and community priorities.

But the core job for health practitioners is to strengthen the hand, and reinforce all the best instincts, of the public sector planners who have the job, through spatial planning, of coordinating and integrating policy in the interests of the whole community, including tackling climate change. They need the help of health professionals!

Climate change, health and planning

Interconnections

Climate change and spatial planning are interconnected on many levels. In terms of combating (or 'mitigating') climate change, planning affects the majority of carbon emissions to some extent: through the energy used in construction, operation of buildings and the transport they generate. It also affects the level of carbon capture and prospects for renewable energy. In terms of coping with (or adapting to) climate change, planning affects the risk of flooding, water supply/use and the temperature of urban areas. This section will deal with each of these in turn.

But first a broader context: spatial planning is one of three key areas affecting the way settlements function to combat and cope with climate change. The other two are technological innovation and changes in values. Technology has to provide part of the answer. The most obvious is in relation to electricity: improved and/or cheaper technologies for capturing renewable energy (not just wind but heat pumps, geothermal, wave, tidal, solar) is critical: it would allow the move to electric vehicles in due course.

Change in societal values is even more fundamental. When people *choose* to act as though the planet matters, then they change the priority they put on, for example, retrofitting their dwelling for energy efficiency or walking short trips.

Spatial planning cannot force changes in these two spheres. But it can act as a prompt, it can open up choices that are currently precluded. It can also be used to block desired change (for example the widespread local political opposition to new wind farms).

Planning and energy efficiency of buildings

Spatial planning, together with building control (often in the same local authority department), have profound effects on the energy efficiency of buildings and therefore on carbon emissions. This is primarily through the progressive winching up of building regulations and the Code for Sustainable Homes (Department for Communities and Local Government, 2008). The government in England and Wales intends all new buildings from 2016 to be 'carbon-neutral', which implies a pattern of localized renewable energy supply for electricity as well as very efficient insulation and ventilation control for heat retention.

The location, design and layout of new building developments can either reinforce or undermine energy efficiency. Almost every aspect is related to it in some way. For example, the orientation of housing affects the ability to collect solar energy. The mix of uses in an area affects the viability of efficient heating and power systems. The location helps determine heat loss and gain.

A closely related sphere, not currently legislated for by the UK Government though equally important, is the amount of energy and materials used in the construction process. This so-called 'embodied energy' is profoundly affected by the density, form and structure of buildings and the efficiency of the infrastructure.

Planning and transport

The other (huge) aspect is transport. Transport energy use accounts for about a quarter of total carbon emissions in the UK (see Chapter 1), and is increasing despite improvements in the efficiency of vehicles. *The trick here is not to think of transport as 'mobility' – that is, people in vehicles able to move freely – but 'accessibility', that is, people able to get to the places they want to go.* It is not just a matter of an efficient road system, or even an efficient and safe walking, cycling and public transport system. It is about the whole shape of the town, the city, the region. Are the places people need/want to get to (offices, shops, schools, surgeries, parks etc.) at the most accessible locations? Are they the appropriate scale to match the needs of users, not just the operational require-ments of providers? It will be obvious to you that the current pattern of cities and regions, geared to car and lorry use, must change.

The climate change mitigation agenda outlined above to reduce energy consumption is powerfully consistent with other health goals: reducing fuel poverty, promoting physical activity, working for social inclusion. Health practi-tioners can strengthen the resolve of the planners and councillors on reducing greenhouse gas emissions by stressing the potential health bonus.

The other mitigation measure to mention is carbon capture. Trees and other flora fix carbon, transferring some of it to the soil over time. So the total amount of tree cover (and both Britain and Ireland are among the least forested lands in Europe) must increase (see Chapter 9 for more on the health and climate change benefits of trees).

Adaptation: Coping with climate change

Turning to coping strategies: these are going to be needed even if we are successful in slowing the pace of climate change (see Chapters 1 and 12). Increased flooding is already with us and in the UK the Environment Agency (responsible for overseeing the resource and environmental issues) has made great play about safeguarding flood plains. But this needs to be seen in the wider context of water management – the whole water cycle. The built environment needs to be designed to allow infiltration of surface water into the ground, recharging aquifers (permeable rock that stores groundwater) and reducing the speed of water run-off into streams and rivers that causes flooding. The threat to coastlines is a more intractable problem: in many situa-tions a managed gradual retreat is the only answer (even when some commu-nities have to be relocated).

The other vital ingredient of a coping strategy concerns the urban landscape. The amount of greenery in a city (and reduction of exposed brick, tarmac, slate and concrete) can lower summer temperatures by several degrees. Urban areas, churning out heat from buildings, factories and vehicles, are typically several degrees hotter than the usual ambient temperature: the urban 'heat island'. As summer overheating becomes more of a problem than winter cold, the greenness of the city increases in health significance: roofs, gardens, streets, parks can all go green, or greener. Again, the incidental health benefits can be emphasized by the health lobby: green landscape is a mood enhancer, giving a sense of well-being and counteracting depression, reducing violence and promoting social cohesion (see Chapters 3 and 4).

So the potential benefits of active involvement in the planning process by health practitioners are considerable. On the one hand the potential health benefits of the combating and coping strategies add weight to the climate change arguments. On the other hand climate change can, ironically, help health organizations deliver on some of their other health goals. In other words we can get potential health benefits, such as more policy emphasis on active travel, on the back of the dominant climate change agenda.

Mechanisms for integration

In the previous section, we saw how spatial development has a profound impact on the wider determinants of health including climate change. The overarching aim for health and sustainable development must be to achieve a 'good fit' between spatial development and all its inevitable impacts on the human and natural systems. A 'good fit' means minimizing adverse and unwanted impacts and maximizing possibilities for human utility and well-being. But how can we do this?

Spatial change is mainly driven though investment in the built environment. Public and private investment attempts to provide social benefits (e.g. social housing, state education facilities, transport routes) and a return for private profit (e.g. speculative office or residential development). The overarching mechanism, mediating between market and public conflict, and bringing governance in the public interest to spatial development, is the spatial planning system. The exact form this takes and the statutory mechanisms involved differ from country to country, but we can identify three distinct mechanisms where we need to act:

- the realm of collaborative partnerships;
- the statutory planning and land use system;
- the processes that are used to evaluate and appraise impact.

Collaborative partnerships

At almost every spatial scale, from national and regional to city and neighbourhood, collaborative partnerships can be found. These partnerships set the strategic direction and agree on the core issues.

Collaborative processes seek to negotiate between disparate interests and align goals between different organizations and/or businesses. Differences in interest are found not only between the private and public sectors, but also within the public sector, comprised as it is of many different agencies, often pulling in different directions. Partnerships seek to articulate a common vision on which joint or individual agency action is then based.

Digging down into these sectoral silos, we often find the fundamental interest is either in people (as consumers, clients or patients) or the environment (in terms of biodiversity, aesthetics or resources). If we approach these collaborations with a health remit, bringing both climate change and health to the table, we can act as enablers: enablers for a consensual vision between them, advocating outcomes that meet both.

Collaborative processes can occur at different spatial scales, for example at regional level and at local level for major neighbourhood or urban regeneration. An example from England, at the municipality level, is the Local Strategic Partnership with its associated Local Area Agreement (similar arrangements exist in Scotland, Wales and Northern Ireland). This collaborative body agrees a document known as the Community Strategy, which sets out a vision, which then becomes the basis for spatial development plans in the statutory planning system (see Box 6.1).

For health practitioners, being active within the Local Strategic Partnership provides membership of a powerful collaboration for tackling the wider determinants of health, including climate change.

Box 6.1
Example: An outline of the basic collaborative structures in England

Local Strategic Partnerships

In England, Local Strategic Partnerships bring together local organizations from the public, private, community and voluntary sector. Working together to improve the quality of life in a neighbourhood, they contribute to the development of Local Area Agreements and community plans. They can play a central role in identifying health improvement initiatives. The purpose of Local Strategic Partnerships is:

- To ensure a Sustainable Community Strategy is produced. This should set the vision and priorities for the area agreed by all parties, including local citizens and businesses, founded on a solid evidence base.
- To be the 'partnership of partnerships' in an area by ensuring strategic coordination and linkage of all local partnerships and other plans and also bodies at regional, subregional and local level.
- To agree and implement a Local Area Agreement (the delivery plan for achieving the Sustainable Community Strategy).

Local Area Agreements

A Local Area Agreement is a three-year contract that sets out priority outcomes for a local area, as agreed between central government and a local area represented by a local authority and Local Strategic Partnership. Local Area Agreements simplify arrangements for utilizing funding streams from central government to achieve locally determined outcomes and improved local service delivery. The aim is to join up public services more effectively, thus allowing greater flexibility for local solutions to local circumstances. Local Area Agreements can thus help to devolve decision-making away from central government and reduce the bureaucracy associated with multiple funding streams and monitoring arrangements.

Local Area Agreements can be effective at spreading health outcomes across non-NHS partners and in making the links between Local Strategic Partnerships and spatial development in the built environment.

Sustainable Community Strategies

The 2006 English Local Government White Paper (Department of Communities and Local Government, 2006) describes their role as follows:

> The role of the Sustainable Community Strategy is to set out the strategic vision for a place. It provides a vehicle for considering and deciding how to address difficult cross-cutting issues such as the economic future of an area, social exclusion and climate change. Building these issues into the community's vision in an integrated way is at the heart of creating sustainable development at the local level.

The Sustainable Community Strategy is prepared by the local authority with the Local Strategic Partnership and in consultation with local people, businesses and community and voluntary groups. The strategy balances and integrates social, environmental and economic needs and goals, based on shared evidence and agreed priorities across the partnership. It must take account of national and regional priorities and integrate with other local plans. The Sustainable Community Strategy should establish long-term goals, but also set short-term priorities for action through the Local Area Agreement.

Statutory planning

The key mechanism in any country for control of spatial development is the national statutory planning system. Although details vary between countries, a system of policy linked together with territorial maps or plans is used to direct and control development and land use. Since this system modifies private property rights over land in the name of public interest, it is very common for there to be several points where developing plans and policies are open for consultation.

What is vital here for health practitioners is an understanding of both the process of planning and the content of the plans. Planning processes can be long and drawn out affairs, since the final development documents may need to guide development for the next five to ten years or longer. There is usually a preparatory phase where data and policies are being drawn up, followed by several consultation stages. Health practitioners, if not engaged already, need to be able to recognize what stage of the planning cycle has been reached and know how to enter the process. If in doubt, we must use local authority planning officers to facilitate our engagement: that is part of their job.

In terms of plan content, it can seem a large leap from the words in a policy and the lines on a map to their potential health and climate change impacts. Depending on the level of plan, we may need to find allies and specialists to help unpick the likely impacts from these quasi-legal and sometimes technical policy documents. For proper health scrutiny, it is important to dig beneath the outward facing 'public' consultation documents, get hold of as much detail as possible and meet with the planning officers who are involved with policy and plan development. We must ensure that adverse impacts on health and, in particular, the wider determinants of health are identified, articulated and fed back into the plan-making process. A good starting point is the 12 key objectives for Healthy Urban Planning (see Table 6.1 below).

Box 6.2
Key elements of the UK planning system

Regional Spatial Strategies: The RSS for each region of the country sets the big agenda in terms of overall priorities, economic development, levels of planned housing provision and the location of future major development.

Local Development Framework: The LDF applies the broad strategy of the RSS at the level of the individual local authority, setting out the policy and spatial framework, through a series of linked documents that may include quite detailed plans and guidelines for specific areas or topics.

Core Strategy: The Core Strategy is the most critical part of the LDF, which deals with the spatial framework – the relationship between transport, land use, environment, social and economic development.

Development Management: This is the statutory process for ensuring that development proposals are consistent with the LDF. It involves planning applications and the development control function of local authorities.

Appraisal in the built environment

A powerful tool in our health toolbox is promoting understanding of the wider determinants of health within the appraisal of built environment policies and plans. Almost every country uses some form of appraisal to assess the impact of interventions in the built environment on specific areas of concern. Confusion reigns, as there are a number of different 'methods', with different names in different countries and with different statutory bases, such as sustainability appraisal, environmental impact assessment, statements and reports and strategic environmental assessment. Let's start with Environmental Impact Assessment; we can then understand the whole field as it relates to this process.

Environmental Impact Assessment (EIA)

This has been defined as 'the process of identifying, predicting, evaluating and mitigating the biophysical, social, and other relevant effects of development proposals prior to major decisions being taken and commitments made' (IAIA, 1999). A European Union directive known as the EIA Directive introduced this into the European Union in 1985. An EIA applies to a known plan or proposal. In Australia and New Zealand the term Environmental Assessment is commonly used.

An EIA is obligatory for some prescribed major or controversial developments (e.g. airports or nuclear power plants). It may be requested by a planning authority in certain other circumstances (e.g. large developments with land reclamation), or even undertaken on a voluntary basis by developers demonstrating good practice in risk mitigation and stakeholder consultation. When undertaken as a statutory requirement the form of an EIA is strictly controlled and this form is often used in other applications.

The parts of the EIA that are of particular interest to public health are:

- The description of the environment. This must list all aspects of the environment that may be affected by the development, for example: human populations, fauna, flora, air, soil and water.
- The description of the significant effects on the environment as described above.

- The mitigation – what is being done to reduce the harmful effects on the environment.
- The non-technical summary – this is referred to as the Environmental Impact Statement (EIS).

Though 'humans' are listed as an 'aspect' of the environment, the full health implications of a development are rarely explored. In particular, the impacts of climate instability and conditions such as obesity should be a focus for health practitioner involvement (see Chapter 4 for a summary of the evidence base).

Strategic Environmental Assessment (SEA)

SEA can be understood best as an EIA but applied to policies or programmes rather than projects. In the EU the so-called Strategic Environmental Assessment (SEA) Directive (2001/42/EC) is now in force. In the UK an assessment called Sustainability Appraisal is applied within the spatial planning process. The basic format and content of the assessment process is similar to that described above for EIA.

Assessing the health impacts of spatial change

In theory EIA and SEA are processes that have the ability to address impacts on the wider determinants of health, though in practice the degree to which they do this depends on the skills and approaches of those undertaking them. Health impact assessment, as a broad approach not a specific named tool, can be used stand-alone or integrated into these comprehensive processes. The important point is to ensure that health impacts are adequately addressed.

Whatever tool is being used, an early stage will be what is referred to as a 'scoping phase'. It is during this phase that issues requiring more detailed impact study are identified. We need to work closely with local authority planners to be alerted at this scoping stage. If we raise health concerns about the proposed policy or plan, backed up with a good basic evidence base, we can have maximum leverage on the subsequent conduct of the study.

Box 6.3
Spatial development and health: Some online evidence and resources

- Sustainable Development Commission: 'Health, place and nature: how outdoor environments influence health and well-being: a knowledge base', available at www.sd-commis sion.org.uk/publications/downloads/Outdoor_environ ments_and_health.pdf (accessed 5 February 2009)
- Glasgow Centre for Population Health: 'Health and the physical characteristics of urban neighbourhoods: a critical literature review', available at www.gcph.co.uk/component/ option,com_docman/task,doc_download/gid,159/ (accessed 5 February 2009)
- Health Scotland, Greenspace Scotland, Scottish Natural Heritage, Institute of Occupational Medicine: 'Health impact assessment of greenspace', available at www. greenspacescotland.org.uk/upload/File/Greenspace%20HIA. pdf (accessed 5 February 2009)

Examples of collaborative approaches

Collaborative approaches to influence spatial development for healthy, sustainable low-carbon communities can take many different forms. The following examples attempt to demonstrate a wide variety of types of collaboration and show the integration of health and planning at its best.

- Freiburg, Germany: Healthy communities supported through putting a high value on both quality of life and quality of the environment.
- World Health Organization Healthy Cities Europe: Cities across Europe bringing health and urban planning practitioners into ever closer alignment.
- London, England: A capital city supporting better public health engagement with the statutory planning system.
- Helsingborg, Sweden: A strategic but practical alliance between health and sustainable development.

Freiburg, Germany

The citizens and municipal authorities in Freiburg, south-west Germany, have held quality of life and environmental quality at the top of their agenda for over 20 years. The outcome has been to change the very culture and behaviour of the population; from car-dominated urban lifestyles to a city with a reputation

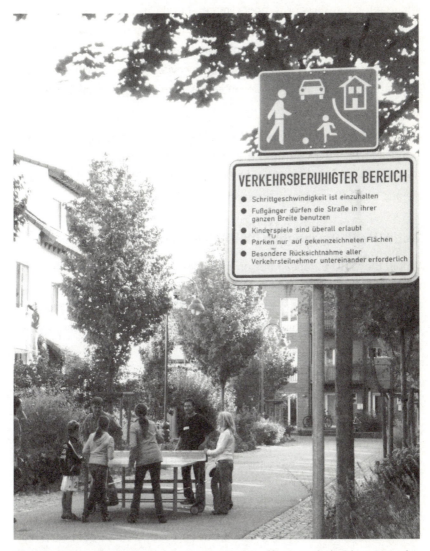

Figure 6.1 Freiburg, Germany: Residential traffic is so light that Saturday morning sees neighbours playing table tennis in their street

Source: Marcus Grant, 2008

for active travel and inclusive public spaces and streets. Over this long times-cale the actual infrastructure of the city has changed to support healthier lives. It is especially evident in the high degree of thought and integration in public transport, leading to very high levels of popular use. The newer suburbs, by design and not by chance, have well-located good local facilities and very low levels of car use leading to streets being reclaimed as social spaces. Equally important for sustainability and climate stability is the profusion of solar panels, sustainable drainage schemes, green roofs, combined heat and power systems and many other technological and design solutions that reduce the negative environmental impact of the built environment. At each step, there is an attempt to create win–win outcomes both for the planet and for the community.

Although there are many elements of context that are unique to Freiburg, we can draw a useful lesson from this case study. That lesson is just how much they have achieved for health and well-being through focusing on quality of life and the local and global environment.

World Health Organization (WHO) Healthy Cities Europe

Within the WHO European Region more than 1200 cities are members of a national network connected to the WHO Healthy Cities. A smaller group of 90 cities more advanced in their Healthy Cities approach are direct members of the WHO Healthy Cities network. The core principles of the Healthy Cities approach are:

- Commitment to the Healthy Cities project at the highest political level of the municipality.
- Creation of organizational structures for implementing the policies within the Healthy Cities project.
- Formulation of a common vision of the city with a focus on public health.
- Formal and informal networking within the Healthy Cities project.

Now in its third decade, the Healthy Cities approach seeks to put health high on the political and social agenda of cities and to build a strong movement for public health at the local level. Emphasis is given to equity, participatory governance, inter-sectoral collaboration and action to address the determinants of health.

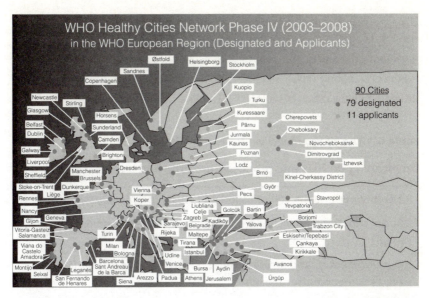

Figure 6.2 The healthy cities network across Europe; many other cities are associated through membership of one of the many national networks

Source: WHO European Region, 2007

Recent Healthy Cities activity has focused on four themes:

- Healthy ageing: to generate strong local political commitment and policies that will ensure a holistic and well-balanced approach to the health and care needs of older people.
- Health impact assessment: to support integrative health impact assessments to enable decision-makers to take account of people's health and well-being.
- Physical activity and active living: to develop strategies and innovative interventions (including changes in urban design and environment) that encourage physical activity for all ages.
- Healthy urban planning: to integrate health considerations into city urban planning programmes and to establish the necessary capacity and political and institutional commitment to achieve this goal.

Cities progressing their Healthy Urban Planning work have been increasingly supporting joint working between planners and public health teams. Collaborative projects have been undertaken at many scales from strategic city planning and policy development to planning frameworks for specific sites, or programmes (e.g. active travel/cycling), to smaller-scale housing and regeneration projects. The cities developed 12 key objectives though their own experiences during Phase 3 (1998–2002), which they have used ever since to promote healthy urban planning:

Table 6.1 The 12 key objectives for Healthy Urban Planning

Do planning policies and proposals promote and encourage:

1 Healthy personal lifestyles, including activity in everyday living?

2 Social cohesion and inclusive communities, the development of social capital?

3 Development of and access to good quality housing at a variety of sizes, tenures and affordability?

4 Access to work?

5 Accessibility to local facilities?

6 Access to good quality food and local food production?

7 Crime reduction and community safety, including freedom from the fear of crime?

8 Equity of access and reduction of inequalities?

9 Air quality, noise reduction and attention to good quality design and aesthetics?

10 Healthy systems for provision of water and sanitation, including reduction of flood risk?

11 Effective use of land and minerals, including waste minimization, recycling and re-use?

12 Climate stability?

Source: Barton and Tsourou (2000)

We can immediately learn from the experience of the European Cities and use these healthy urban planning objectives in our own localities. For example, in London they were used as the basis for the 'Watch out for health!' checklist (see below).

London, England

In 2004 the 'NHS London Healthy Urban Development Unit' (HUDU) was established. HUDU's role is to help the National Health Service engage and be proactive in relation to the health and planning agenda for London. It does this through supporting the 31 NHS Primary Care Trusts (health service commissioners) across London. It is funded by these 31 trusts and the London planning authority.

HUDU aims to improve communication and cooperation between the spatial planning and health sectors in London in order to: 'respond to the capital's unique mix of challenges in terms of population change, development pressures, environmental constraints and the delivery of healthcare services' (HUDU, 2009).

The staff can work closely with the Primary Care Trusts and planning authorities where needed, but have developed a number of generic tools:

- 'Watch out for Health': based on the WHO Healthy Urban Planning Objectives (see above), this tool takes these further, adapting them for use in London and embedding the list within a set of working guidelines. Its aim is to help health practitioners to influence planning proposals to maximize the benefit to human health and enable development proposals to be justified for their positive effect on health.
- 'Delivering Healthier Communities in London': this document provides evidence linking public health issues and spatial planning and examples of how health issues can be addressed through the planning process. It aims to ensure that health is sufficiently taken into consideration when spatial plans are formulated.
- 'Health and Urban Planning Toolkit': this document sets out a systematic approach to building the relationship between Primary Care Trusts and Local Planning Authorities. It is a handbook on how the Local Development Framework and planning application process should address health.

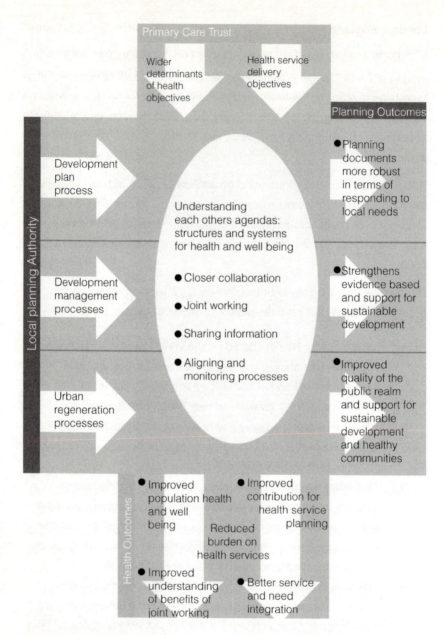

Figure 6.3 Summary of interactions between Primary Care Trusts and Local Planning Authorities

Source: Healthy Urban Development Unit (2007) p66

HUDU have also developed a tool for calculating the additional health service demands that will be generated by a housing proposal, enabling health service providers to argue for a contribution to these costs from the developer. The planning system in the UK supports a legal process for such contributions.

The lesson we should take from this approach is that having a dedicated team of planners, working for public health within the statutory planning system, is starting to pay rich dividends for health. In real monetary value, the tool to enable health service providers to obtain a contribution from developers to additional health service costs has alone enabled health services to claim substantial funding from developers. Moreover, in starting to turn the tide away from development that can literally make communities sick, HUDU's tools are making clear to a wide audience the links between 'good' planning and healthy communities.

Helsingborg, Sweden

Helsingborg has been a member of the WHO European Healthy Cities Network since 1999. Their Healthy Cities project has focused on public health and sustainable development and has developed a collaborative approach expressed in the 'Plan for Sustainable Development'. It has seven improvement areas for Helsingborg: work and education; conditions during childhood and adolescence; housing and urban development; health and living habits; healthy ageing; environmental quality; and safety and security. All these areas are linked through carefully developed health and sustainable development objectives. There is commitment to the collaboration between health and sustainable development at the highest political level. The Plan for Sustainable Development is one of four strategic documents of the municipality adopted as a basis for financial planning.

In Helsingborg there has been a change within municipal activity from focusing on minor projects to a mainstreamed method. The concept of sustainable development has broadened from a concern for the environment to include all three perspectives (social, environmental and economic). When interviewed, municipal officers gave housing, work and education as examples of areas for fertile cross-working between public health and sustainable development (Municipal Executive Council's Delegation for Sustainable Development, 2007).

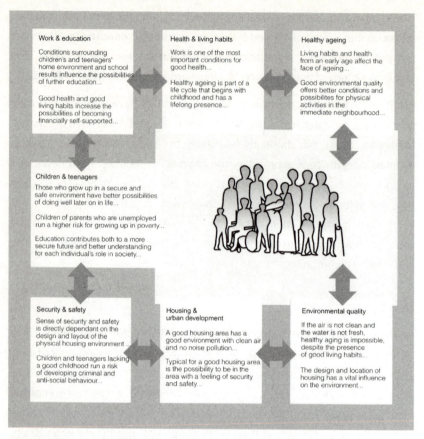

Figure 6.4 The web of health and sustainable development

Source: Municipal Executive Council's Delegation for Sustainable Development (2007).

The work in Helsingborg validates the rationale underlying this book: that there is great strength in the synergy between health and sustainable development.

Neighbourhood planning

We now focus on more specific areas of policy: first, the neighbourhood.

There is a real need for health practitioners to make their priorities clear to designers, land use planners, transport planners and regeneration leaders involved in both new development and gradual retrofit of existing neighbourhoods. All the elements of the climate change strategy, outlined earlier in this chapter, come together at the neighbourhood level. Recent research suggests that work at this level may well be more important than strategic/regional planning in combating climate change (SOLUTIONS, 2009).

What the health agenda does is to strengthen the arguments for a new direction. Reducing transport emissions, promoting physical activity, creating a socially inclusive, convivial, supportive environment, all pull together towards an integrated pedestrian-centred vision of neighbourhoods.

The question, though, is how to get involved? When health practitioners are working in a particular community it is appropriate to try to influence things at that level. There may be opportunities if major developments (regeneration, 'brownfield' or 'greenfield' sites) are in the offing and the developers or the local authority launch a participatory process. (The term 'brownfield' site refers to land that is or was occupied by a permanent structure, which has become vacant or derelict and has the potential for redevelopment. 'Greenfield' land is a catch-all term for land that falls outside the planning definition of previously developed land, it may have current agricultural uses, be a woodland or even a derelict airfield.)

But there is a danger in getting dragged in to local politics too deeply – you may lose much time and confuse your role. If possible try to avoid engaging with policy detail or very specific proposals. The built environment professionals are paid to get that right. It is normally better to be 'strategic', spotting the key documents and meetings where it would be helpful to respond or to stand up and talk, and addressing the fundamental strategic and design objectives. That means making sure you are on the consultation list, but not worrying about trying to get on top of all the documents. They are often difficult to interpret for a non-expert and might bog you down.

It is much more important simply to state and restate the health priorities, linking them where possible to other local concerns and to the wider agenda of climate change. The objective is to impress people (residents, councillors and professionals alike) with the importance of the health agenda and to build networks of support, making allies who can then amplify your message because they see it as being in their own interest.

Of course there may be occasions when the health organization has resources to throw at a problem – perhaps a major redevelopment of a socially deprived area with poor health status. In these situations partnership is the key. An alliance should be formed with the local authority, which needs the help and support that the health organization can provide. The quid quo pro is that health and climate change objectives must go into the starting brief of the project. *Nothing is more important!* If the original objectives are right, and understood, then the chance of a good outcome is hugely increased. Conversely if they are weak, then no amount of later remonstration or health impact assessments will compensate. The objectives need to be 'bought into' by all the major players. Then the art is to carry them though into the appraisal of the area, the options considered and the refinement and implementation of the final strategy. The health representatives can act like a kind of watchdog for this process, checking consistency, supporting dialogue when the inevitable conflicts emerge, brokering partnerships and nudging towards health objectives when necessary.

The assessment processes described earlier in the chapter are very useful. Assessment does not have to take the form of a Health Impact Assessment. It may take the form of a 'sustainability appraisal' or 'integrated appraisal'. But it does need to include climate change and other health criteria quite explicitly. The two essential ingredients of success are that:

- Assessment on health criteria works right through the planning process, starting with the initial objectives, not just coming in at the end of the process when often it is too late.
- It involves all the main stakeholders, including the local community. For example, one such process – known as 'Spectrum' – talks about 'inclusive rationality' (Barton and Grant, 2008).

Where major change is not afoot, involvement at the local level may not be appropriate. However, there are always incremental changes going on that may exacerbate or help manage climate change and car dependency. These will be guided by the contents of the Local Development Framework that covers the whole local authority area (see earlier). So it is action at that level that is important. The health organization, as part of the Local Strategic Partnership (in the UK) must try to ensure that the right objectives get in at the start: through the Community Strategy and the Core Strategy. Perhaps even more important than the documents themselves are the key people. *It is vital to reach, and convince, the movers and shakers.* This includes the politicians and chief officers on the one hand, but also the major investing companies, through their chief executives.

In other words it is rather pointless going to long and tedious meetings, wrestling over the wording of a strategic document, if at the same time there is not support and networking at the highest level. The devil will only be in the detail if the power brokers give the 'wrong' signals to drafters. Look therefore to befriend and inspire the leaders. Be a champion for healthy, sustainable communities! (For more ideas on taking action in your community, see Chapter 9.)

Transport and accessibility

Sustainable transport is an exceptional example of policy synergy. Measures to reduce carbon emissions (transport is responsible for a quarter of all carbon emissions in the UK) by promoting a shift from the car to the lowest-emission forms of transport – walking and cycling – also encourage physical activity, reduce road casualties, cut local toxic air pollution, improve the aesthetic quality of the public areas in our communities and, by bringing people on to the streets, help to address anti-social behaviour (see Chapter 4 for more information). The benefits are felt in so many policy fields, so widely across society and in areas of such intense official focus, that it may be useful to pause and consider why more is not yet being done to roll back the dominance of private motor transport.

A key factor is that policy-makers and planners in transport, land use and development control suffer from the 'windscreen perspective'. Historically, people in these roles have tended to be motorists with quite complicated working and travel lives. They tend to assume that everyone else lives a similar life and – probably not intentionally – have created transport systems that favour the car. Even in the case of policies and measures intended to promote reductions in private motor transport, it is noticeable that officials focus these on travel to work. In fact, the lifestyles of planners and managers are non-representative of society as a whole, as Figure 6.5 shows. It comes from the detailed study of

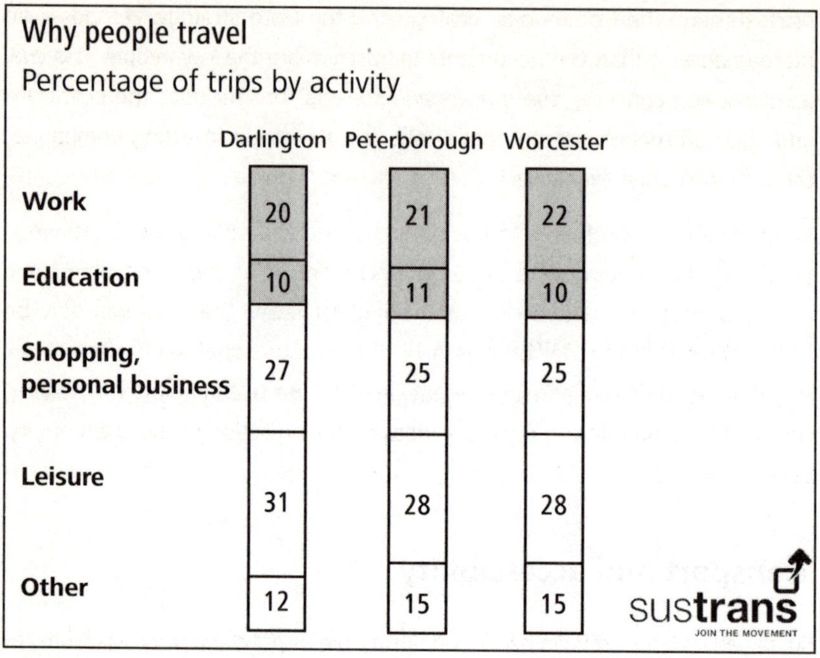

Why people travel
Percentage of trips by activity

	Darlington	Peterborough	Worcester
Work	20	21	22
Education	10	11	10
Shopping, personal business	27	25	25
Leisure	31	28	28
Other	12	15	15

sustrans
JOIN THE MOVEMENT

Figure 6.5 Why people travel: Percentage of trips by activity

Source: Sustrans and Socialdata (2005)

trip choices and travel behaviour undertaken in three English towns in 2004 and shows the breakdown of trips within the town boundaries. Only one in five trips are work-related and over a half are for shopping, personal business and leisure.

This is also likely to be true of policy-makers and programme managers in the health sector, and indeed we have seen the unedifying spectacle in the UK of NHS bodies lobbying against the Edinburgh congestion charge proposals and professional associations demanding free car parking at hospitals. We all of us need to take care that our personal preferences and concerns do not interfere with good, health-focused decision-making based on evidence and good practice.

The good news is that in the transport field, policies from a range of sources all tell us the same thing: we need to restrain and restrict private motor transport, take road space from the car and work to create environments that actively encourage walking and cycling. Health policy tells us this is an effective way to promote active living; transport policy may still focus on the dubious objective of congestion reduction but confirms the message; new planning guidance (as we have seen) seeks the social benefits and for climate change policy – reducing carbon emissions – the benefits are obvious. The health practitioner can – and should – work across all the sectors involved to ensure that strategies and plans relating to transport do, in fact, reduce our reliance on private motorized transport.

Mobility versus accessibility

If we are to promote significant behaviour change in transport, we need to change the way spatial planners and transport strategists have viewed transport since the end of the Second World War. Until very recently, *mobility* has been viewed as good in itself and the ability to travel further and faster as innately desirable. This is now changing, and today's thinking is that mobility is the sacrifice we have to make in order to reach the goods, services and experiences we desire and that what we actually need is *access*.

The mobility approach was to build bigger motorways, larger car parks and urban distributor roads almost irrespective of what had to be demolished to do so. The outcome – predictably – was increasing centralization of services, the demise of much local business and ever-longer trip lengths.

Accessibility demands that we localize as much as possible, make walking and cycling routes shorter, quicker and more attractive than those for motor traffic and take back some of the advantages we have handed to the car. Effective planning for accessibility will see us switch many car journeys to walking and cycling and to public transport; it will also see us travelling less, because we no longer need to make so many and such long trips.

The potential for change

The two main problems facing society that can be addressed by a move to sustainable transport are carbon emissions and ill health caused by sedentary living. Both are immense in scale and demand change on a transformational level in the way we live our lives. It is therefore important to look at the potential for travel behaviour change and consider how much benefit we could gain from effective intervention.

Constants in travel behaviour

Daily mobility	On average, people make three trips per day, spending one hour travelling
Activities	Only one in five trips is work-related
Spatial orientation	Five out of six trips begin or end at home
Car trips	10% are not further than 1km, 30% are not further than 3km and 50% are not further than 5km

Socialdata

sus**trans**
JOIN THE MOVEMENT

Figure 6.6 Constants in travel behaviour

Source: Sustrans and Socialdata (2005)

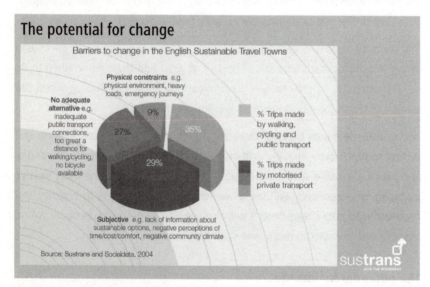

Figure 6.7 The potential for change

Source: Sustrans and Socialdata (2005)

Travel behaviour research across the developed world shows considerable constancy in the trips people make and how they make them. Averaged across the whole population, people make 1000 trips a year, five out of six of which begin or end at home – in other words, most trips are simple origin to destination journeys and do not form part of a complex 'trip chain' that might make behaviour change more complicated. And, looking for a moment at car trips, one in ten is under a kilometre, 30 per cent under 3km and 50 per cent under 5km (see Figure 6.6). There is clearly significant potential for a modal shift to more benign travel.

In 2005, as part of the Department for Transport's Sustainable Travel Demonstration Towns programme, Sustrans and Socialdata looked more intensively at travel behaviour in Darlington, Peterborough and Worcester (see Figure 6.7). Over 1200 participants were asked about the factors surrounding every trip they made over a week – journey purpose, whom they travelled with, weather, loads to be transported, availability of bike or car. This information and the choices they made were checked against external determining factors of which the respondents might not be aware, such as public transport services. In brief, the researchers found that 35 per cent of trips within the three towns were made by walking, cycling and public transport; the remainder by private motorized transport. But of these 65 per cent, almost half could easily and realistically have been made by at least one other, more benign, mode. The factors preventing people from making wiser mode choices were mainly information-based (respondents were unaware of public transport services or the existence of bike routes) and perceptual (many respondents systematically overestimate public transport cost and travel time, and underestimate these for their car).

The potential for a shift to low-emission and healthy travel revealed by these studies is immense. It would be possibly virtually to double people's use of walking, cycling and public transport *without making significant change to the environment*. The reallocation of road space from private motor transport, traffic calming and other measures now advocated by so many instruments of policy offer still further potential.

The health practitioner should ensure that colleagues in planning and transport departments are actually aware of this potential and that they are seeking to capture it – and directly advocate for it themselves. If your work involves health education or health promotion (as a general practitioner or a health trainer, for example), or if you coordinate programmes on physical activity, healthy walking etc., you could make a big difference to both health and carbon emissions by telling your patients and clients, as well as local authority contacts, about the importance of practical measures to promote more walking and cycling and reduce car use. Refer also to Chapter 9 on action in the community for more ideas.

Public opinion

Media debate regarding transport policy is dominated by a vociferous motoring lobby, which cares little for sustainable development or public health. It seems that media professionals may also suffer from the 'windscreen perspective' – strident comment from motoring campaign groups is often accepted as being representative of the wider public view.

But it is not representative and when communities are asked, they express strong preference for healthier and more sustainable transport. In a 2008 study in Exeter, Lowestoft and Watford, Sustrans and Socialdata found that 87 per cent of respondents think traffic has increased, 83 per cent view this increase negatively and nine out of ten consider sustainable transport to be a priority for planners and policy-makers (Sustrans and Socialdata, 2008).

Transport, energy security and cost

There is one other factor we should not overlook in considering transport, sustainability and health: we are now at the end of the era of cheap energy. This book is not the place to discuss the shocks predicted for individuals and society as energy prices rise and supply continuity is damaged over the coming years. However, each cloud may have a silver lining and we can be confident that these circumstances will drive future transport policy away from the emphasis on motorized mobility. As increasingly sedentary living has been an unintended consequence of the move to motorization, so the balance of advantage must inevitably shift towards healthy, active travel. The challenge for health practitioners will be to contribute to steering this shift, so that the environments we create for the future are as satisfying, attractive and health promoting as possible.

If you are in the UK and wish to advocate for improvements for healthier, low-carbon travel policy, you may want to look at the recommendations in a policy call produced jointly by the Association of Directors of Public Health and Sustrans. 'Take action on active travel' is endorsed (at the time of writing) by 91 health environment and transport organizations (ADPH and Sustrans, 2009).

There is information on travel planning and workplace health in Chapter 10, which focuses on action in organizations, and on travel behaviour change using social marketing approaches in Chapter 8. In partnership with other organizations, Sustrans and Socialdata have pioneered the 'TravelSmart' approach in the UK. If you live in Australia, the United States, Canada, Germany, Austria, Switzerland or France, you may already know about the TravelSmart way of encouraging more walking, cycling and use of public transport through Individualized Travel Marketing, as TravelSmart has targeted more than 3 million people across these countries (Sustrans, 2008).

An end to fuel poverty

In cold climates, improving the insulation and heating efficiency of homes is another excellent example of policy synergy that can improve health and lower carbon emissions. Fuel poverty is defined as the need to spend 10 per cent or more of disposable income to achieve adequate warmth. It is estimated that 3.5 million households experience fuel poverty in the UK. It is associated with low incomes, poor insulation and heating systems and under-occupation of houses, particularly by older people living alone. The health consequences are considerable, both in terms of excess winter deaths and hospitalization for illnesses related to the cold (Department for Business Enterprise and Regulatory Reform, 2008). Cold is associated with increased risk of heart attacks and strokes, respiratory illness, risk of falls and mental health problems.

In the UK, help to install improved heating, insulation and draught-proofing is available through the government's 'Warm Front' scheme in England (Department for Business Enterprise and Regulatory Reform, 2008) and similar schemes in other UK countries. Assistance reduces both carbon emissions and expenditure on energy, thus taking people out of fuel poverty with climate benefit. 'Warm Front' has found that the most vulnerable are least likely to respond to traditional marketing methods. Word of mouth recommendations and reassurance from trusted sources such as health practitioners are vital. Opportunities for reducing health inequalities are being missed, as those with less health needs take up grants.

There is a reduction in carbon dioxide emissions in the average household that has received help from the government's 'Warm Front' scheme of 1.3 tonnes per year (an 11.5 per cent reduction), while helping to achieve affordable warmth. Although referrals from health agencies to 'Warm Front' have increased recently, health practitioners are urged to publicize it and related schemes to tackle fuel poverty and reduce carbon emissions at every opportunity.

Action points

1   How would you adapt the '12 key objectives for healthy urban planning' for your own area of work? What would you need to add/emphasize? What might you leave out?

2   Can you identify the key plans and forums where climate change is being addressed by your local authority? In the UK, the plans are likely to include the Regional Spatial Strategy and the Core Strategy at the least. The most important forum may be the Local Strategic Partnership. Find out what is going on also in relation to regeneration, housing, transport, economic development, neighbourhoods, new urban extensions etc.

3   Can you establish what stage the policy-making has reached and make contact with key policy-makers and conveners to register your interest and potential involvement? Identify the opportunities for involvement at the level of basic objectives and policy – health input can be much more influential at this stage than after completed plans are circulated for consultation.

4   Can you find the time to review the relationship between climate change and health (as described in this book) and prepare a briefing document for your department or directorate to demonstrate the need to be involved at the highest level? Highlight the potential synergies between a strategy to combat and cope with climate change and strategies to combat obesity, health inequalities, air pollution and to promote mental well-being.

5 Can you identify other groups and individuals with related interests and build alliances with them, so that your message is amplified when you are not present? For example, the health inequalities agenda and the social inclusion agendas are mutually reinforcing; bodies concerned with the quality of the environment, or active local campaign groups such as those addressing cycling, may find your arguments help their case.

6 Think about how you can ensure that subsequent participation in spatial policy is at the highest level when priorities are being set, and that it is maintained at an intermediate level with a watching brief, always focusing on the objectives and principles that inform the policy documents and evaluation processes, and emphasizing the potentially huge health benefits of effective action on climate change.

7 What tactics can you use to reach, and convince, the movers and shakers? This includes politicians and chief officers, but also the major investing companies, through their chief executives.

8 Seek to ensure that spatial and transport planning professionals are aware of the wealth of official guidance that now directs them to create walkable and cyclable environments rather than prioritizing motor traffic. Some useful documents are listed in the resources section at the end of the book.

9 How can you inform decision-makers and colleagues about the research, reviewed in this chapter, that shows that people tend to systematically overestimate public transport cost and travel time and underestimate these for their car; and that it would be possible virtually to double people's use of walking, cycling and public transport *without making significant change to the environment*, with the right support for behaviour change.

References

ADPH and Sustrans (2009) 'Take Action on Active Travel' available at www.adph.org.uk/downloads/policies/Take_action_on_active_travel_2009.pdf (accessed 7 February 2009)

Barton, H. and Grant, M. (2008) 'Testing time for sustainability and health; striving for inclusive rationality in project appraisal', *The Journal of the Royal Society for the Promotion of Health*, vol 128, no 3, pp130–139

Barton, H. and Tsourou, C. (2000) *Healthy Urban Planning*, Spon Press, London, on behalf of the World Health Organization

Department for Business Enterprise and Regulatory Reform (2008) 'The UK Fuel Poverty Strategy, 6th Annual Progress Report 2008', available at www.berr.gov.uk/files/file48036.pdf (accessed 7 February 2009)

Department of Communities and Local Government (2006) 'Strong and Prosperous Communities – The Local Government White Paper', available at www.communities.gov.uk/publications/localgovernment/strongprosperous (accessed 5 February 2009)

Department for Communities and Local Government (2008) 'The Code for Sustainable Homes', available at www.communities.gov.uk/documents/planningandbuilding/pdf/codesustainhomesstandard.pdf (accessed 4 February 2009)

HUDU (2007) 'Healthy Urban Planning Toolkit', NHS Healthy Urban Development Unit, London

HUDU (2009) available at www.healthyurbandevelopment.nhs.uk (accessed 7 February 2009)

IAIA (1999) Principles of Environmental Impact Assessment Best Practice, available at www.iaia.org/modx/assets/files/Principles%20of%20IA_web.pdf (accessed 5 February 2009)

Municipal Executive Council's Delegation for Sustainable Development (2007) 'Plan for sustainable development in Helsingborg 2007', Department for Sustainable Development, Municipal Executive Council, Helsingborg, Sweden

Office of the Deputy Prime Minister (now Department of Communities and Local Government) (2005) Planning Policy Statement 1: Delivering Sustainable Development (PPS1), available at www.communities.gov.uk/publications/planningandbuilding/planningpolicystatement1 (accessed 4 February 2009)

SOLUTIONS (2009) 'Final Report of the EPSRC SOLUTIONS Project Consortium' (Sustainability of Land Use and Transport in Outer Neighbourhoods), forthcoming, available at www.suburbansolutions.ac.uk (accessed 11 February 2009)

Sustrans (2008) 'Leading the way in travel behaviour change', Information Sheet FF36, Sustrans 2008, available at www.sustrans.org.uk/assets/files/travelsmart/behaviour_change_ff36.pdf (accessed 11 February 2009)

Sustrans and Socialdata (2005) 'Travel Behaviour Research Baseline Survey 2004: Sustainable Travel Demonstration Towns', Sustrans, Bristol, available at www.sustrans.org.uk/assets/files/travelsmart/STDT%20Research%20FINAL.pdf (accessed 7 February 2009)

Sustrans and Socialdata (2008) 'Nine out of ten people see sustainable transport as a priority', *The Network*, Winter 2008, p19, available at www.sustrans.org.uk/assets/files/Publications/Sustrans_theNetwork_issue09.pdf (accessed 11 February 2009)

World Commission on Environment and Development (1987) 'Our Common Future', the Brundtland Report, Oxford University Press, Oxford

7 How You Can Make a Real Difference

Lindsey Stewart and Alan Maryon-Davis

Be the change you want to see in the world.

Mahatma Gandhi

Summary

I will if you will ... people are more likely to change their behaviour if they see others are doing it too, making them feel that their efforts are worthwhile. It just needs that first step, or the second or even the third, and the aim of this chapter is to give you a helping hand along the way. We take you through how to get a better understanding of your carbon footprint and then offer you lots of practical tips on how you can reduce your domestic energy consumption, drive down your travel carbon emissions, save carbon on your food and drink and reduce waste. You will save money, you will be healthier and your quality of life will be better. Health practitioners can be exemplars within the growing movement of people worldwide living the low-carbon, healthy lifestyle that is so much more fulfilling and rewarding. By doing so, because you are a health practitioner, you will have a huge impact on wider public and political attitudes and behaviour. Though we have based our descriptions on the carbon footprint of people in the United Kingdom, we hope that readers in other countries can easily adapt the suggestions to their own circumstances.

Key terms

Carbon footprint: The amount of carbon emitted by an individual (or a family, town, country), usually measured as kilograms or tonnes of CO_2e released. Carbon is becoming a currency and the carbon costs of our activities are being identified.

Excuses, excuses

No doubt you are well used to seeing headlines about climate change and its effects: melting polar ice caps, desertification in sub-Saharan Africa, sweltering heatwaves in Europe, the devastation caused by hurricane Katrina (and we hope you have read all about it in Chapters 1 and 2 of this book).

If you accept that climate change and its accompanying events and disasters are at least partly human-made, you might be tempted to think that it is too late now to do anything about the problem. Climate change is inevitable and that's that. There's absolutely no point in trying to head it off. It is as futile as King Canute raising his hand to stem the rising tide.

Then again, perhaps you are prepared to believe that something could be done to reduce global warming – but only if all the big industrial nations take determined collective action at government level to reduce their carbon emissions. Smaller countries like the UK are merely bit players and nothing we might do would make any meaningful difference. So why should we bother?

Or perhaps you fully accept that climate change is a massively important issue that must be tackled by every nation, large and small – but that it is really all about macro government-level policies dealing with power stations, transport and procurement rather than the puny efforts of individuals switching to low-energy lightbulbs and using the bike instead of the car.

Wrong, wrong, wrong and wrong. Some global warming is now inevitable, but there is still time to prevent or ameliorate the worst effects of it. Concerted action is certainly needed by governments across the globe, but one way to help make that happen is for countries held in high regard to set an example and lead the way. All nations are made up of communities and communities are made up of individual people. Change comes through a combination of top-down and bottom-up approaches.

As this book argues from start to finish, health practitioners are especially well placed to make a real difference: by advocating low-carbon local policies, by influencing the decision-makers in health care services, by providing appropriate lifestyle advice to patients and by setting an example in their own private lives.

Whichever country you work in, and at whatever level in the system, as a health practitioner you are in a privileged and powerful position to help shape people's habits and the way things are done. Health professionals are widely trusted. Our advice tends to be heeded. But to be credible we have to set our own house in order. We have to be exemplars. We need to practise what we preach.

This chapter is a mini-guide to the many ways in which you personally can contribute to the collective effort of health practitioners throughout the world to combat global warming by reducing not just your own and your family's carbon footprint, but also by using your example and your influence to reduce the carbon emissions of your patients, workmates, workplace, local community and even your national government.

'I will if you will'

People are more likely to change their behaviour if they see others are doing it too, making them feel that their efforts are worthwhile – the 'I will, if you will' approach. By helping to make a low-carbon lifestyle more the norm – indeed the 'cool' thing to do – we can help to consign to history all those gas-guzzling 4x4s and all that food that has travelled halfway round the world. But someone needs to make the first move to get the momentum going, to show it can be done. This is why health practitioners have such a vital role.

If you work in the health sector you can see first hand the effects that a lack of action on climate change has on the physical and mental health of those who use your services – respiratory disease from air pollution; obesity as a consequence of little physical exercise and ill health as a consequence of poorly

Box 7.1

Why people don't adopt more 'sustainable' behaviours

- We are creatures of habit, reluctant to make changes that challenge our routines.
- We are highly influenced by the social norms we see around us.
- We often lack access to facilities like good public transport or doorstep recycling.
- We perceive sustainable options to be expensive and niche.
- We are pre-occupied with short-term household budgets and, for low-income consumers, making ends meet on a weekly basis.
- We often do not trust the government bodies and businesses that are exhorting or enticing us to change.

Source: Sustainable Consumption Roundtable (2006)

designed homes that leak energy and money leading to fuel poverty (see Chapter 4 for the health benefits of acting on climate change).

Whatever your reason for picking up this book, this chapter will show you that taking action on climate change as an individual is just as important as international agreements – perhaps even more so. Governments, especially politicians, do eventually respond to public opinion and habits. If each of us takes action, our collective effort will snowball into a major movement that will actually encourage and empower our governments to be serious about cutting carbon. Not just hot air and hollow targets – but real change.

They will if you will!

Box 7.2
Why should I?

Q. *What's the point of me doing something if most other people won't?*

A. Think of any great social movement – civil rights, women's liberation, football – and you'll find it began with a small number of committed enthusiasts who acted as the spark for change. You can help spearhead the low-carbon movement in your workplace or neighbourhood. If you do it, others will follow.

Q. *But what about the government? And countries like the USA and China that go on pumping out vast amounts of CO_2?*

A. By taking action ourselves we are, in effect, demonstrating our willingness for government to take action, to mandate on our behalf and put pressure on the big CO_2-polluting countries to 'green-up their act.'

Q. *How much can I save by going low carbon?*

A. Loads. Think of all your electricity, gas, heating oil, petrol or diesel bills. You can seriously reduce them by just turning appliances off, not leaving them on standby and turning your heating down by just a few degrees. For example, swapping just one light bulb to a low-energy light bulb can save you £60 a year.

Q. *Why is the low-carbon life good for my health?*

A. Active travel, like walking or cycling, is good for your heart and circulation, your general fitness and your well-being. Cutting down on red meat and replacing it with poultry, fish, grains, pulses or vegetables (preferably locally sourced) will be good for your health (particularly your heart and your waistline) as well as the environment. If you are not convinced, have another look at Chapter 4.

Q. *I'm a health professional. As well as making changes to my own lifestyle, how can I encourage my patients/clients to do the same?*

A. Always ask your patients/clients about their activity level, or their diet, or what kind of heating they have at home. Mention your own lifestyle changes. And then get them to commit themselves to their own carbon-cutting programme.

Q. *How long have we got before things get really serious?*

A. They already are! Some experts have calculated that we have less than ten years before we hit the tipping point of 2°C. That is when irreversible and catastrophic impacts kick in. But there is a lot we can do to lessen the impact – as long as we start *now*.

Q. *My friends and I feel it is hopeless – too little, too late. We are in despair.*

A. We still have just about enough time to stop runaway climate change, if we get on with it. We can create a social movement. There are lots of people out there giving it a go – find some of them in your communities or professional networks. We must show future generations that we tried – see the examples in Chapter 9.

Q. *OK, I am ready to make the change to a healthy, sustainable, low-carbon lifestyle. How do I go about it?*

A. Read on – fast!

First things first

Know your own carbon footprint

Even if you are already recycling your household waste, switching to low-energy light bulbs and making less use of the car, it is a good idea to work out what your carbon footprint is. This will give you a baseline against which to check your progress. When you are well on the way to your low-carbon lifestyle, it will be good to look back at that original footprint and see just how far you have come.

Setting a baseline can also show you where your biggest impact is. For example, you might think it is that long-haul flight you took for your holiday. But it actually turns out to be the joint of meat you put in your shopping basket every week. Red meat not only takes a huge amount of energy to produce, but it might also have travelled thousands of miles before it got to your dinner table (see Chapter 4).

At about 10 tonnes of CO_2 per person, the UK is about halfway up the international league table for carbon emissions. We have a smaller per capita footprint than Ireland, Germany, Estonia or Greece. Top is Qatar (69 tonnes) – second is Kuwait (38 tonnes). The US average is 24 tonnes. For a league table of carbon emissions in different countries and continents (and a reference to look up if you want), have another look at Chapter 1.

Figure 7.1 shows how the average person's 10 tonne CO_2 footprint is made up in the United Kingdom (figures are in metric tonnes, i.e. 1000kg).

So, we know is the average carbon output of the average person in the UK. But what about you? You might not fly all that much, you might not own a car. Or you might have a five-bedroom house that uses a lot of gas and electricity. How do you know exactly where your CO_2 emissions are from and, more importantly, how can you work out where you need to cut the carbon?

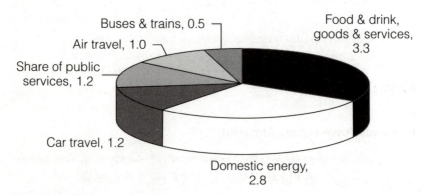

Figure 7.1 Where the average UK individual's carbon footprint comes from, in tonnes per person per year

Source: Griffiths and Stewart (2009)

How to add it all up

The best way to work out your own personal carbon footprint is by using a 'carbon calculator'. These are, primarily, online tools that ask you various questions about certain aspects of your life such as how you heat your home or how often you travel by car or fly, in order to help you tot up the total. Useful calculators include:

- Act on CO_2: http://actonco2.direct.gov.uk/
  This has been set up by the UK Government and allows you to measure your home energy usage, appliances and transport. It will also provide an action plan with tips on how and where to reduce your carbon emissions.
- World Wildlife Fund: http://footprint.wwf.org.uk/
  As well as energy usage and travel, this calculator also counts if you have a pet. In addition to your carbon footprint, it will also tell you what your ecological footprint is.
- My Carbon Footprint: www.mycarbonfootprint.eu/
  The European Union's calculator takes a slightly different approach from the other two above. It calculates how much carbon you can save by making the changes you are willing to make.
- Chris Goodall's book *How to Live a Low-carbon Life* (2007) is a reference guide to calculating and reducing your CO_2 emissions, as a recommended alternative to websites.

Our rough-and-ready-reckoner

These online calculators are quite sophisticated and thorough. But if you just want a rough estimate to get you started, here is our very simple ready-reckoner based on the main categories in the UK piechart above.

Domestic energy use

- **Electricity and gas**

  Find your last few electricity bills and check your quarterly usage in kilowatt-hours (kWh). Add up the total kWh for your household over the past year.

Total household electricity usage = xxx kWh

Now divide this by the number of people in your household, including babies and children. (Yes – even babies have a carbon footprint – and it's not as small as you might think.)

Assuming that each person has an equal share of the electricity usage…

Your share of the electricity is = yyykWh

Now multiply this by 0.43 to convert it to carbon emissions in kilograms (kg)

Your carbon footprint for electricity is yyy × 0.43 = zzzkg

Now do the same for your gas usage. Your gas bills give a quarterly figure in kWh equivalents (ignore the gas 'units'). Work out your share of the annual household gas usage in kWh equivalents and multiply this figure by a conversion factor of 0.19 to get your carbon footprint in kg:

Your carbon footprint for gas = qqqkg

- **Other forms of heating**

  If you have oil-fired central heating, or use a coal or wood fire to heat your home, do the following sums along the lines we used for electricity and gas.

  - *Heating oil*: Work out your share of the litres of oil in the past year and multiply by 3.0 to get your oil carbon footprint in kg.
  - *Coal*: This is the least green fossil fuel. Multiply your share of the weight burned (in kg) by a factor of 2.0 to get your coal carbon footprint in kg.
  - *Wood*: By contrast, this is a renewable source of energy, and is effectively carbon neutral. Burning wood produces CO_2 – but this is equal to the CO_2 absorbed from the atmosphere by the trees that produced the wood in the first place. In other words, there is no net addition of CO_2 to the atmosphere and it does not add to your carbon footprint.

Transport

- **By car**

  Your car's footprint will vary according to engine size, fuel type, miles per gallon of fuel and mileage travelled. Look up your car's emissions in grams per kilometre (g/km). If it's not in the owner's handbook you can search for the figure on the internet (the UK Government's Act on CO_2 website has some information).

  Multiply the emission figure by the number of kilometres driven in a year (km/y = mileage x 1.6). Divide this total by 1000 to get your car's annual CO_2 emissions in kg.
  Now estimate how much of the car use is down to you personally. Decide on a percentage and apply it to the subtotal:
  Total personal car footprint = ???kg
  (You can use a similar calculation if you drive a motorbike or scooter.)
  Within the UK, as a rough rule of thumb, travelling alone by car is about twice as carbon-intensive as going by train or bus. But the real baddie is flying – about *five times* as carbon-intensive as taking the train or bus.

- **By train or bus**

  Broadly speaking, buses and trains have more or less the same carbon footprint per head per mile (at least for shorter journeys, though high-speed long-distance trains emit more carbon than coaches). Work out your average weekly mileage and convert it to kilometres by multiplying by 1.6, and then multiply by 52 to get your annual distance travelled. Now divide this figure by 10 to estimate the carbon cost in kilograms:
  Total bus/train footprint =XXXkg

- **By air**

  Calculating the carbon cost of a plane journey involves a similar formula to car travel – but obtaining the figures is a lot more complicated – not least because planes vary in their passenger capacity and fill rate, and because the extra fuel needed for take-off and landing makes short-haul flights relatively more carbon-intensive per passenger mile than longer flights. The easiest way to reach the answer is to use an online flight carbon calculator (e.g. www.chooseclimate.org). Using London as a case study, Table 7.1 shows the carbon cost of some popular international return flights.

Table 7.1 The approximate CO_2 equivalent costs of some popular international return flights from London

These CO_2 equivalents (see Chapter 1, 'Key terms' for definition) include a multiplier (×3) to account for the additional warming effect of high altitude emissions.

Destination	Approximate kg CO_2e
Paris	740
Dublin	580
Nice	920
Rome	1210
Malaga	1400
Athens	1780
Dubai	4110
New York	3490
Antigua	4630
Nairobi	4750
Mumbai	4890
Los Angeles	5930
Tokyo	6550
Cape Town	6250
Sydney	11,090
Auckland	12,020

Source: www.chooseclimate.org/flying/mapcalc.html

Add together all the flights you've taken in the past year:

Total flying footprint =XXXkg

Now add up all your transport totals – car/motorbike, bus/train and plane – to reach an overall total for transport.

Total transport total = YYYkg

General consumption level

This is the roughest and readiest estimate of all – because to calculate accurately the carbon cost of all your food and drink, goods and services and share of public infrastructure, would be a quite a challenge. But here are three very simple ballpark categories to choose from. Which one fits you best?

- **Carefree consumer**
  You like to indulge yourself – within reason of course. You love the latest fashions, luxury items or high-tech gadgets. You eat more or less what you like, you love red meat and never worry about 'food miles'. Your annual consumption footprint is about 4500kg.
- **Middle-of-the-road consumer**
  Apart from the occasional splashing out, you are fairly modest in your consumer choices. You shop 'sensibly' and usually only buy things you need. You buy most of your food once a week at the supermarket and keep a keen eye on the prices. Your annual consumption footprint is about 3000kg.
- **Lean and green consumer**
  You like to lead a rather frugal existence – the 'good life' – as self-sufficient and planet-friendly as you can. You would rather mend things or have them repaired than throw them away and replace them. You look for food that is in season or grown locally. You are an arch recycler. Your annual consumption footprint is about 1500kg.

Totting it all up

Finally, add your totals together – domestic energy, transport and general consumption. Add another 1200kg for your share of public services such as schools, the National Health Service, the local council and the myriad of other goodies that our taxes provide. And hey presto! – you have arrived at your very own Grand Total Personal Carbon Footprint.

Now, divide this by 1000 to convert it into tonnes and compare it with the UK average (about 10 tonnes). Are you higher or lower? To put your score into perspective, the average person's CO_2e footprint in the US is 24 tonnes; in China, 4 tonnes; in India 1.5 tonnes (see Table 1.1 in Chapter 1). The footprint of people in some sub-Saharan African countries is one or two tenths of a tonne.

In the next section we outline some of the key areas where, by making simple changes, you can make some really substantial carbon savings.

How to cut your carbon – and help save the planet

You've done your carbon calculation, you know your footprint. What then can you do to reduce your emissions? The answer is: plenty. In this section we will be concentrating on those main areas where emissions tend to be highest:

- energy use;
- travel;
- food;
- general consumption and waste.

Domestic energy use

As we saw in Figure 7.1, the average person in the UK emits almost three tonnes of CO_2 from domestic energy use alone: heating, lighting, household appliances. You can do a lot to use your household energy more efficiently – and not only cut the carbon but also save the money.

Have a look at the energy-saving checklist below. The calculations are based on a three-bedroom, semi-detached house. Financial savings, quoted in pounds sterling, are for illustrative purposes only. The principle of financial and carbon savings will generally hold true whichever country you live in.

Energy-saving checklist

- Switch to energy-saving light bulbs: one 20 watt energy-saving light bulb (equivalent to a 100 watt ordinary bulb) can save as much as £60 over its lifetime and 172kg of CO_2 each year.

- Turn off appliances and lights: leaving televisions, computers and other equipment on standby can cost you up to £40 and emit almost 160kg of CO_2 each year.
- Wash your clothes at 30°C or lower: it uses less energy than a hotter wash and your clothes will be just as clean.
- Turn down your thermostat: for every 1°C you lower your thermostat you will not only cut your carbon emissions by an average of 330kg per year but it could also save you a tidy sum on your heating bill. (But, vulnerable people such as older people, people with ill health and young children are at risk from the cold. Seek further advice if you are uncertain.)
- Don't hesitate – insulate: insulating walls, floors, loft space, tanks, pipework and windows (e.g. double glazing) could give you a massive annual saving of almost £550 and save an enormous 4380kg of CO_2. (Grants for some of the cost may be available from local or national government.)
- Install energy-saving appliances: you could save £100 per year and 430kg of CO_2 by using only those appliances (such as fridge-freezers, washing machines) that have the highest energy-efficiency ratings. For UK rating and European Union rating information, see www.energy.eu/#saving. For US appliance rating information, see http://apps1.eere.energy.gov/consumer/your_home/appliances/index.cfm/mytopic=10030
Installing a condensing boiler with heating controls can also save you a further £270 and over 1700kg in CO_2.
- Switch to a 'green energy' provider: one that uses renewable sources such as solar, wind and wave energy.
- Generate your own energy: solar panels for hot water or even solar photovoltaic cells, mini-wind turbines and ground source heat pumps are just some of the ways you can produce your own energy. In some areas, it may be possible to develop a community energy generation scheme.

Table 7.2 Home energy – less carbon, lower bills

Illustrative carbon and cost savings on energy for the average United Kingdom household per year (2008 prices)

Change	Carbon saving	Cost saving
Energy-saving light bulbs (assuming 6 per house)	1032kg	£36
Switching off standby equipment and lights	160kg	£40
Turning down the central heating thermostat	260kg per 1°C	£35
Proper insulation throughout	4380kg	£550
Converting to energy-efficient appliances	430kg	£100
Changing to a 'green' electricity provider	800kg	–
Solar water heating	250kg	£100

Travel

All in all, transport accounts for over a quarter of the average UK resident's carbon footprint, with the car taking the lion's share. Our dependency on those four wheels accounts for 12 per cent of our total carbon emissions. If we really want to cut our carbon, many of us will have to radically rethink how we get around. Fortunately, there are lots of greener ways to travel.

Greener travel checklist

- Walk or cycle: rather than driving, walk or cycle whenever and wherever you can. Not only will it cut carbon emissions (and air pollution), it is also good for both your physical and mental health and well-being. And of course you will also save money on fuel.
- Use public transport: if you need to travel then wherever possible take the bus or the train instead of driving your car. On average, using public transport is about half as carbon-intensive per person mile as going by car.

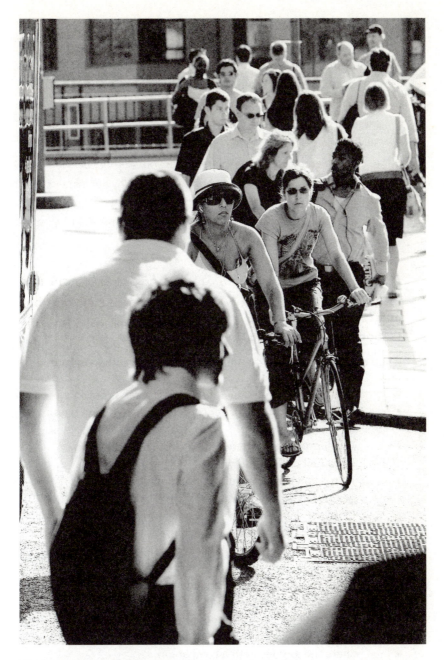

Figure 7.2 Commuters: Bristol Bridge/Castle Park
Source: J. Bewley/Sustrans

- Try to avoid flying: especially short-haul air travel, which has a disproportionate effect on the environment compared to long-haul flights (Department for Transport, 2004). Take the train in the UK and to Europe and instead of connecting flights. On average, flying is about five times as carbon-intensive per person per mile as taking the train or bus.

- Share your car journey: if you have no alternative to going by car, try to find a friend to share the journey with you. Another person in the car can almost halve the carbon footprint. Why not join or start a car-sharing scheme?

- Try tele- or videoconferencing: instead of travelling to meetings. It could save you valuable time and money.

Box 7.3
Carbon-conscious driving

If you really must use the car, here's how to cut its carbon output:

- Drive as small and as energy-efficient a car as possible.
- Slow down: you use 25 per cent less fuel at 50mph than at 70mph.
- Accelerate gently: roaring away from the lights burns extra fuel unnecessarily.
- Turn down the air conditioning: it uses electricity generated by the engine.
- Close the windows (especially when driving at higher speeds) to reduce drag and save fuel.
- Remove the roof-rack when not in use, again to reduce drag.
- Lighten the load: keep luggage to a minimum and empty your car boot; the more weight, the more fuel.
- Keep tyres properly inflated: for every 6psi that a tyre is under-inflated, fuel consumption increases by 1 per cent.
- Share the journey with a companion.

Source: Griffiths and Stewart (2009)

Other reasons to think about giving up your car, apart from reducing carbon emissions.

'What if giving up your car was to make your life better? What if being car-free meant being richer, thinner, fitter, saved your time, maybe saved your life, and was better for your kids? When there weren't many of them, cars were quick and convenient. Now, they are becoming a bit of a nightmare, what with the traffic jams and the road rage and the parking problems. Cars eat up your time. In fact, the total costs of car ownership outweigh the benefits ...'

This is from http://GiveUpYourCar.com.

Food and drink

Stop and think about the food you put in your supermarket trolley. Where did it come from? How much carbon was spent getting it to you? Will all of it be consumed before the sell-by date? How much food do you generally throw away each week? How much of it goes straight in the bin, or do you compost it?

For the average UK household with children, the cost of wasted food is over £600 a year (WRAP, 2008). Nationally it amounts to an annual carbon footprint the same size as the entire National Health Service – a whopping 18 million tonnes of CO_2! By only buying what we need, including in restaurants, and carefully storing our food we can not only save carbon but also money.

Food and drink carbon-saving checklist

- Cut down your 'food miles': so many of the perishable foods in our supermarkets are flown in from far-flung places across the globe. Check the labels. Those green beans might have come from Egypt, Ethiopia or Ecuador; the prawns from Honduras or the North Atlantic. Think of the energy (and carbon emissions) it has taken to get these products to your shopping basket.
- Buy more fresh, local produce in season: fewer food miles, less energy spent on storage, more jobs for local people. If you must choose all-year-round products – like bananas or coffee – always look for the fair-trade version.

- Reduce your consumption of animal products (meat and dairy): livestock production is responsible for 9 per cent of all 'human-made' carbon dioxide emissions, 18 per cent of all greenhouse gas emissions and 37 per cent of all methane associated with human activity (Food and Agricultural Organization, 2006, see also Chapter 4 for more information). Cutting down on your consumption of animal products is also better for your health (as you will cut down your intake of saturated fat). The increasing industrialization of livestock production also has welfare implications for animals.
- Don't waste food: buy (or order in restaurants) only what you need (see Box 7.4).
- Grow your own fruit and vegetables: you don't need much space; just a plant pot on a window ledge or a bucket full of soil could give you a decent crop of tomatoes or potatoes.
- Try to avoid drinking bottled water: tap water in the UK has one of the highest standards of quality. Bottled water has huge environmental costs – from the use of plastic bottles to the costs of transportation and landfill or recycling. And of course, tap water is excellent value for money.

Box 7.4
Want not, waste not

It's a staggering thought but *every day*, the UK throws away:

- 5.1 million potatoes;
- 4.4 million apples;
- 2.8 million tomatoes;
- 7 million slices of bread;
- 1.3 million unopened yoghurts;
- 1.2 million sausages;
- 1 million slices of ham;
- 700,000 whole eggs.

This equates to 6.7 million tonnes of food each year, of which 340,000 tonnes is still in date. A further 1.2 million tonnes is simply food we leave uneaten on our plates.

Source: WRAP (2008)

Box 7.5

Case study: The Fife Diet

The Fife Diet asks people to sign-up to eating food from Fife for a year, monitor their progress and share their experience. This is a celebration of local goodness not an exercise in self-denial. Like many other regions, Fife has loads of fruit and vegetables, excellent farm-reared lamb, beef, poultry and an abundance of seafood. The project was inspired by Vancouver's '100 Mile Diet' (http://100milediet.org) and aims to bring people together who want to prepare for a low-carbon future.

Source: http://fifediet.wordpress.com/about/

Reducing waste

Between them, the EU-15 countries produce almost two billion tonnes of waste each year, of which 335 million tonnes comes from the UK (Defra, 2006a). Over 70 per cent of UK waste still goes to landfill producing almost one million tonnes of methane (Economic and Social Research Council, 2008; Defra, 2009). Household levels of recycling are increasing (though the UK still lags behind some of its European counterparts) but we still send nearly 29 million tonnes of rubbish to landfill (Defra, 2006b). You can do your bit by sticking to the three 'green' Rs: *reduce, reuse, recycle.* Here are some tips on how.

Less waste checklist

- Buy less – of everything. Become a leaner, greener, less-consuming consumer. Perhaps this is not exactly 'on message' when we are supposed to be spending our way out of global recession. But if we all consumed less of modern life's non-essentials we could strike a real blow for a more sustainable planet. And when you do buy something, make sure it is as energy-efficient and eco-friendly as possible, especially electrical goods. And ask your supplier to recycle your old equipment. (You will also save money.)

- Compost as much as you can – as well as green garden and kitchen waste, you can also compost teabags, eggshells, shredded newspaper, and even vacuum dust.
- Recycle – if you cannot compost it or give it away, then recycle it. Although recycling consumes energy, it is still better than sending things to landfill.
- Get a water butt – climate change brings hotter summer weather so store rainfall for use on the garden during dry spells.
- Join in or start up a recycling scheme in your local area. Swap things you no longer want with people who do.

Other action you might want to take...

- Spread the word: get your family and friends involved. Generate some friendly competition – see who can recycle most in the week etc. Tell your colleagues at work. If you will, they will! If you're a health practitioner, there's plenty you can do to encourage others – see the case studies below and check out the other chapters in Part II of this book.
- Get involved in local green initiatives: there are lots of groups out there involved in making their local environment a nicer, more eco-friendly place to live. And as well as improving the environment, you'll meet lots of new people, find out more about your local neighbourhood and get fit in the process. Check out your local library/community centre or search online. And see Chapter 9 for ideas.
- Write to your local MP: ask them what they're doing on your behalf on climate change.

And if you feel really, really ambitious...

- Galvanize action in your local community: start a local carbon reduction group; if you have children or are a teacher, encourage your school to be a healthy/eco school (if they are not already; if they are, get involved). You could even encourage your local area to become a Transition Town (www.transitiontowns.org). And check out Chapter 9 focusing on community action on climate change,

which has lots more on Transition Towns and other community
initiatives.

Health practitioner case studies

Here are three case studies of health practitioners: a general medical practitioner, a health visitor (a community health promotion nurse) and a public
health trainee. The case studies are intended to stimulate thought and debate.
What more could these people do to make a real difference to driving down
carbon emissions and improving people's health while they do so?

Case study: Dr S, general medical practitioner

Dr S is lives in an average, three-bedroom, semi-detached house with her
husband and two children. Dr S drives 11 miles to her surgery, first dropping
off the children at their local school (just under a mile away). They take a two-
week family holiday in the summer, usually in Europe (which they fly to). The
family tries to recycle as much as they can, they have installed energy-efficient
light bulbs throughout their home and have double glazing and insulation. So
what else could they do? Here is Dr S's top tip tick list:

- Holiday closer to home – or take the train or ferry to Europe rather
  than fly.
- Check whether the school organizes a local school bus or, even
  better, a 'walking bus scheme' where children walk to school
  (supervised by parents) – it is good for their health. If they do not,
  suggest they do.
- Talk to patients about ways they can improve their health (such as
  walking to the surgery, if they are able to, or improve their diet –
  more fruit and vegetables, less meat) and reduce their carbon
  emissions.
- Buy seasonal, locally produced products, or better still, grow her
  own fruit and vegetables – the whole family can join in and it will
  give Dr S's children a better understanding of where their food
  comes from.
- Talk to colleagues and see how the surgery itself can reduce its
  carbon footprint and become a 'green surgery' (see Chapters 10
  and 11).

Go through the checklists in this chapter and see how many others she can tick.

Case study: Ms Y, health visitor

Ms Y is a health visitor. With two children both at nursery – one of whom is under a year old – she needs her car not only to get her round the village but also to take her two children to nursery (there is only a limited bus service). She lives in a modest terraced house on the edge of the village. She holidays generally in the UK as she can drive and finds it easier than travelling in Europe with her young children. The house is mid-terrace and double glazed. She uses reusable nappies rather than disposable ones for her baby. Top tips for Ms Y include:

- Ms Y's car is essential to her work but if she follows the recommendations in 'Carbon-conscious driving' (see Box 7.3) she could cut her fuel costs and help the environment. She could also write to her local MP and ask them what they plan to do about the poor bus service.
- Check whether her nursery also uses reusable nappies – if not, give them a supply to use throughout the day. Her local council may offer incentive schemes (such as vouchers and cashback) to encourage people to use reusable nappies (rather than disposable ones).
- Check whether there is sufficient loft insulation – although a mid-terrace house will get heat from those houses on either side, heat is lost through the roof. It will save her money (and carbon emissions) in the long term. She might also be eligible for grant funding if offered by her local/national government.
- When going on holiday, try taking the train or coach rather than driving.
- When visiting patients/clients, share health messages and assess them for risk of fuel poverty (see Chapter 6 and Smith and Edmondson-Jones, 2006 for more information on fuel poverty, health and carbon emissions). If visiting new mothers, encourage the use of reusable nappies rather than disposable ones. Tailor particular messages for each client.

Go through the checklists in this chapter and see how many others she can tick.

Case study: Mr P, public health trainee

Mr P is a trainee public health specialist. He lives in a flat-share in the centre of a large city. He travels to work via public transport. As his flat is in a block, he has no garden and there is little facility for recycling or composting food waste. His flat is rented and he therefore has little leeway in making alterations to the property. However, there are still things that Mr P can do to reduce his carbon emissions:

- Switch to a green energy supplier: this is not generally dependent on the landlord.
- Install energy-efficient light bulbs: they last longer, will save Mr P money and use less energy.
- Pool resources with other residents: if there are local recycling facilities nearby, take it in turns to take things for recycling.
- Join a local conservation group and help look after the local environment.
- If he has a warm window ledge, Mr P could try growing herbs or tomatoes. Or join with other residents and get an allotment so he can grow his own.
- Talk to his local deanery (public health training organization) and ask for action on climate change to be included in the training curriculum.
- Talk to colleagues at work: ask for action on climate change to be included in organizational goals and business plans (see Chapters 10 and 11).

Go through the checklists in this chapter and see how many others he can tick.

Towards a low-carbon future

Looking at the simple suggestions laid out in this chapter, it is not so difficult to envisage a future where health and well-being are paramount and low-carbon living is the norm (Griffiths, 2008, personal communication, see also Chapter 6). Here is how things might change – but of course we should not wait until then to take action:

- Each of us will have an individual carbon allowance (a bit like points on a card) that we will trade in, rather like the petrol rationing we had during the oil crisis in the 1970s.
- Fuel, goods and services will bear a carbon tax, like value-added tax (VAT), passed on to the end-user. The effect will be to discourage consumption, and hence provision, of higher carbon items and encourage greener hoices.
- Communities will be developed around pedestrians, cyclists and integrated public transport rather than the car. Money previously invested in road-building programmes will be invested in improving and expanding the public transport infrastructure and routes for walkers and cyclists.
- All new houses, public buildings and commercial buildings will be carbon-neutral. Existing buildings will be retrofitted to improve their energy efficiency and reduce their carbon footprint.
- Community energy generation will be part of our lives, generating collective excitement and interest in how much power can be produced locally.
- Carbon-emitting cars will be a thing of the past – new cars will be powered through renewable sources.
- Flying will be reduced to essential or occasional journeys only – largely replaced by videoconferencing. Companies will wish to be seen as eco-friendly by cutting right down on executive flights. Flights will be taxed more heavily and people will take their overseas holidays closer to home.

Doesn't it sound wonderful? Quality of life could be assured, not just our own but that of the millions of people worldwide who are most at risk of the effects of climate change, as well as that of future generations – if we each of us just take that brave step and let go of our carbon-dependent, carbon-addicted lifestyles. Yes we can – it just needs a willingness to change.

And if you will, the others will.

Action Points

1   Despite the enormity of the global challenge, indeed because of it, what do you think is the true significance of our own individual contribution to the collective effort, especially as health practitioners? What we have going for us as a community and a movement are dedication, a commitment to health and health care and sheer numbers. Working together we amount to an incredibly powerful force.

2   Can you find the time very soon, indeed perhaps now, to review the checklists we have given throughout this chapter and the links we have made with other chapters in Part II and reflect on what steps you can take to make a difference?

3   Can you get started now? What can you do straight away? Can you make a firm commitment to further changes or initiatives as soon as possible?

4   Can you spread the word – and the deed? Encourage family, friends and workmates to join in this powerful movement to save the planet and protect the health and well-being of future generations.

References

Defra (2006a) 'Key Facts about Waste and Recycling', available at www.defra.gov.uk/environment/statistics/waste/kf/wrkf13.htm (accessed 17 February 2009)

Defra (2006b) 'Municipal Waste Management Statistics', available at www.defra.gov.uk/environment/statistics/wastats/bulletin06.htm (accessed 17 February 2009)

Defra (2009) 'E-digest Statistics About Climate Change', available at www.defra.gov.uk/environment/statistics/globatmos/gagccukem.htm (accessed 17 February 2009)

Department for Transport (2004) 'Aviation and global warming', available at www.dft.gov.uk/about/strategy/whitepapers/air/docs/iationandglobalwarmingreport.pdf

Economic and Social Research Council (2008) 'Waste fact sheet', available at www.esrcsocietytoday.ac.uk/ESRCInfoCentre/facts/index29.aspx?ComponentId=7104&SourcePageId=13176 (accessed 17 February 2009)

Food and Agricultural Organization (2006) 'Livestock's long shadow: Environmental issues and options', Food and Agricultural Organization, Rome, available at ftp://ftp.fao.org/docrep/fao/010/a0701e/a0701e00.pdf (accessed 17 February 2009)

Goodall, C. (2007) *How to Live a Low-carbon Life: the individual's guide to stopping climate change*, Earthscan, London

Griffiths, J. and Stewart, L. (2009) *Sustaining a Healthy Future: taking action on climate change*, 2nd edition, Faculty of Public Health and NHS Sustainable Development Unit, London

Smith, M. and Edmondson-Jones, P. (2004, updated 2006) *Fuel Poverty and Health*, Faculty of Public Health, London

Sustainable Consumption Roundtable (2006) 'I will if you will: towards sustainable consumption', National Consumer Council and Sustainable Development Commission, London

WRAP (2008) 'The Food We Waste', available at www.wrap.org.uk/retail/case_studies_research/report_the_food_we.html (accessed 17 February 2009)

8 How to Help People to Change Behaviour

Lucy Reynolds and Allison Thorpe

Knowing is not enough, we must apply.
Willing is not enough, we must do.

Johan Wolfgang von Goethe, 1749–1832

Summary

This chapter provides an introduction to social marketing as a means of helping people to live healthier, low-carbon lifestyles, using a case study to illustrate key learning points. Social marketing aims to understand why people behave as they do (their circumstances, beliefs, physical environment) and to use this understanding to develop a package of support and incentives that will help them to change their behaviour. We have chosen as an example a large-scale social marketing programme about travel behaviour. However, social marketing can also be done on a shoestring. Key principles, tools and techniques are identified that we can all use to inform our work and our interactions with others in daily life. This chapter should give you an understanding of the ways in which you can apply specific techniques to increase the salience of your pro-environmental, pro-health behaviour interventions to your target audience/ customer, and thus increase their effectiveness.

Key terms

Social marketing: The systematic application of marketing, alongside other concepts and techniques, to achieve specific behavioural goals, for a social good.

Customer understanding: The development of a broad and robust understanding of the 'customer' that focuses on understanding their lives in the round, and not only a single aspect or feature.

Segmentation: Identification of distinct sub-groups (segments) that may have similar needs, attitudes and behaviours, using psycho-graphic data as a starting point for developing tailored interventions.

Methods mix: The range of approaches that could help achieve and sustain particular behaviours, aiming to get the optimum mix for greatest potential effect.

Competition: The recognition that whatever is being 'offered' will always face competition, from direct countermessages or simply competition for the time and attention of the same target audience.

Introduction: Why social marketing?

We live in an information-rich society where most people are bombarded by messages from multiple directions and sources and, in many cases, with competing agendas. Assailing people with a white noise of messages in this way is like expecting them to navigate their car on a foggy night on an unfamiliar road – the landmarks obscure, the route unclear and no obvious direction to guide them.

In the climate change and health field, the evidence base is often presented in a highly scientific manner, aiming to give people 'hard facts' (as we do in Part I of this book). However, such an information-intensive approach may actually cause alienation rather than action. By bombarding people with complex information, and emphasizing the consequences of failure on a global scale, we may, inadvertently, be increasing the very barriers we wish to overcome, disempowering people from engaging fully in pro-environmental behaviours.

Preceding chapters have illustrated people's differing levels of awareness of and attitudes to climate change and its consequences. Some people and organizations do not yet fully comprehend the seriousness and urgency of climate change: many social interests conspire to 'manufacture uncertainty' (see Chapter 5). But opinion surveys suggest that many people certainly do now understand. Some are long-standing champions who are very active themselves and perhaps also in their communities and organizations. Others who understand all too well are overwhelmed by a sense of hopelessness – the challenge is too big, we shall never be able to reduce greenhouse gas emissions by such a large proportion in so short a time. They can find the hope they need and deserve by linking up with others who are working at all levels to create a better future, as we suggest throughout this book.

But many others remain non-committal or are stuck in outright denial. Why? Is there something fundamentally flawed about the way we have communicated the information that shapes public perceptions? And if so, what can we do about it?

One reason for some people's inertia might be a lack of clarity about what we are actually asking people to do. By just relaying general information, communication can obscure the importance of individual action. In contrast, social marketing moves beyond fact-based information-giving. It aims to understand what governs behaviour (people's circumstances, beliefs, physical environment) and to use this understanding to develop a package of support and incentives that will help them to change their behaviour. This chapter suggests that social marketing should be considered as part of your arsenal, enabling you to understand the factors that influence behaviour, and to engage more effectively with your key target audiences.

The example of social marketing we use throughout this chapter is 'Choose How You Move' from the city of Worcester in England. The Sustainable Travel Demonstration Towns was an England-wide programme, of which three were funded by the Department for Transport: Worcester, Peterborough and Darlington (see Chapter 6 for more information on sustainable travel). The Worcester programme was city-wide and had a relatively large budget. It used the Sustrans/Socialdata Individualized Travel Marketing package, known as TravelSmart, but under Worcester's overarching 'Choose How You Move' brand.

However, social marketing *can* be done on a shoestring and whether working on a large or a small scale, the same basic principles apply: understand your 'customer', adapt and respond to their needs and don't just *tell* them what to do – help them to actually do it.

We know the sorts of behaviours we need to target (see Chapter 7 for more information). For example, the English Department of the Environment, Food and Rural Affairs (Defra) identified 12 headline behavioural goals, which would substantially reduce carbon emissions and also improve health (see Box 8.1).

Box 8.1
Twelve behavioural goals for reducing greenhouse gas emissions

Home:
1   Install insulation products
2   Better energy management and usage (lower temperatures, turning off appliances)
3   Install domestic micro-generation through renewables
4   Increase recycling and segregation
5   Buy energy-efficient products
6   Reduce consumption of water

Food:
7   Waste less food
8   Eat food that is local and in season
9   Adopt diet with lower carbon emissions (more vegetables, less meat and processed food)

Travel:
10   Use car less and not for short trips of less than three miles
11   Buy or use more energy-efficient, low carbon, vehicles
12   Reduce non-essential flying, especially short haul

Source: Adapted from Defra (2008)

Defra's report (2008, Chapter 3, pp25–25) suggests that focusing on these 12 behaviours will reduce confusion caused by conflicting messages and allow baselines to be set against which progress can be mapped.

Research commissioned by Defra, 'Driving Public Behaviours for Sustainable Lifestyles' (2004), examines the role of habit as a potential barrier to behaviour change. As outlined by Kolmuss and Agyeman in 'Mind the gap' (2002), habit (or 'old behaviour patterns') is the biggest barrier between intention and eventual action. Many of the everyday behaviours outlined above (e.g. turning off the lights or tap) occur at relatively low levels of consciousness. We are often scarcely even aware that we are undertaking these behaviours, let alone considering their environmental impact.

However, habits *can* be raised in profile and subjected to scrutiny in such a way as to catalyse behavioural change. The Global Action Plan (GAP) EcoTeams described in Chapter 9 enable people to scrutinize low-level actions during the course of the programme and then change these patterns before reinserting them into the fabric of daily, habitual life. The aim is to expose a detrimental habit (e.g. leaving the lights on) and to replace it with a positive habit (e.g. always switching the lights off).

This can work effectively where the required changes are relatively small. However, habits prove harder to break when big changes are required and a sacrifice is seen to be necessary (e.g. taking the bus not the car). Social marketing shows that even large behavioural change can be achieved if we can unlock the link between the habit and the action and understand the causes of specific behavioural patterns. It thus offers a much-needed tool for understanding habitual behaviours, breaking the chain of habit and making uncomfortable or effortful changes as easy as possible to achieve.

Using social marketing to address climate change and improve health: A practical guide to changing behaviours

So what is social marketing?

As a health practitioner, you may already have come across 'social marketing' as an increasingly popular approach to changing people's health-related behaviours. The Department of Health (DH) in England has been a forerunner in promoting it (DH, 2004), founding the National Social Marketing Centre in 2006 and adopting social marketing to underpin its own national strategies and local delivery systems across a wide range of priority health areas, including smoking, obesity, alcohol and sexual health (DH, 2008).

Social marketing is not only a health-related discipline. You can think of it as a set of project management principles that can be applied to any programme that aims to understand people and their existing behaviour patterns and then to develop interventions and support that will enable them to change. This is not new learning – although it has been far from systematically applied.

Box 8.2
Worcester Choose How You Move: Introduction

In 2004, the Department for Transport selected Worcester as one of three government-funded Sustainable Travel Demonstration Towns to test out new ways of reducing the impact of personal travel. The findings are being used to inform future UK transport policy.

Results are encouraging: by the end of phase 2 in 2008, 54 per cent of residents contacted by travel experts had requested personalized support packages. Amongst those who received individualized travel marketing, the following behaviour change was recorded over the course of a year:

- Walking: number of trips increased by 19 per cent.
- Cycling: number of trips increased by 30 per cent.
- Public transport: number of trips increased by 13 per cent.
- Car use: single occupancy use declined by 12 per cent.

Sources: Full case example: www.nsmcentre.org.uk; research documents and 'Choose How You Move' website: www.worcestershire.gov.uk/chym/

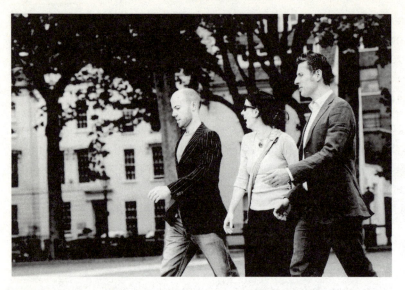

Figure 8.1 Take the scenic commute: Walking through green city square

Source: J. Bewley/Sustrans

Key features of social marketing

The key features of social marketing are described by the National Social Marketing Centre as 'benchmark criteria' to promote consistent delivery (www.nsmcentre.org.uk). These eight criteria offer you a checklist to help you to understand social marketing and how you might try it for yourself.

1 Get to know your customer: 'Customer orientation'

Social marketing builds from the user's perspective. We can use our increasingly sophisticated understanding of what motivates people to develop tailored solutions based on their attitudes, needs and values. We can support people rather than hector them.

By using a mix of quantitative (e.g. statistics) and qualitative (e.g. focus groups) research techniques, you will be able to build a detailed picture about the people you will be working with:

- their existing circumstances, attitudes, beliefs and aspirations;
- their current and the desired behaviours;
- approaches that might be effective in achieving behaviour change.

It is not enough to know about one or two aspects of people's lives or behaviour. Social marketing commits to a thorough front-end research process, using the widest possible range of research methodologies (including desk research, statistical analysis, surveys, expert consultation, focus groups and face-to-face interviews).

As a social marketer, you will develop a deep understanding of what motivates your target audience based on your research and you will use this to underpin the development of your programme. This can help you to identify what might work and to reject what has already been shown not to. Next, you will drill down from your broad understanding, to identify key factors that will be relevant in influencing a particular behaviour.

Box 8.3
Worcester Choose How You Move: 'Customer Orientation'

In autumn 2004, Worcester began a comprehensive research programme to establish existing travel behaviours and identify options for promoting change. Research was carried out by Socialdata and Sustrans:

- postal survey of 4125 people across Worcester's 15 urban wards (some followed up by telephone calls);
- focus groups with school students and teachers, residents and employers;
- smaller in-depth survey and face-to-face interviews.

Further desk research was then conducted, looking at best practice sites in Belgium, America and Australia, to learn from existing programmes.

2 Get to know your customer: 'Insight'

The next benchmark criterion, 'insight', takes us from general information to 'actionable insights'.

You might want to think about how you would use some of these insights, and what practical responses they suggest.

Box 8.4
Worcester Choose How You Move: 'Insight'

The following insights were identified during Worcester's research process:

- 46 per cent of car journeys could be switched to walking, cycling or public transport. (This was calculated using data on a number of factors including trip distance; availability of public transport alternatives; needing to carry large or heavy luggage. These trips were, in other words, being made for subjective reasons which we might expect to be able to influence through social marketing.)
- Major barriers to using public transport were lack of information and poor perceptions of the service.
- People overestimated journey times for public transport by more than 60 per cent, and underestimated car journey times by 20 per cent.
- The majority of people would consider using alternative transport, but did not know how to do so.
- People were making more journeys by sustainable transport than had been expected.

---

3 Use of behavioural theories

Whilst seeking to understand their customer, social marketers consult behavioural theories, which is the next social marketing benchmark criterion. This might sound daunting, so it can help to remember that 'theory is just the distillation of previous work in a particular field: it enables us to learn from experience' (Hastings, 2007, p19).

By looking at behavioural theories, social marketers can understand 'why people act in certain ways, what factors are acting to influence these behaviours and what factors may be amenable to change' (Glanz et al, 2002). They can then develop interventions based on this understanding.

You might want to think about some of these stages and what they mean in reality. If you were designing 'Choose How You Move', what would you do for 'pre-contemplators' and for those 'taking action'? How might the support you offer differ?

Box 8.5
Worcester Choose How You Move: 'Theory'

This recognizes that people have different levels of motivation to change and outlines five stages that individuals go through when adopting a new behaviour:

- Pre-contemplation: an individual does not even consider the behaviour (e.g. taking the bus just isn't an option).
- Contemplation: an individual gains understanding and considers changing. They may seek information (e.g. a person notices a bus timetable and flicks through it to see which routes they might use).
- Preparation: an individual reaffirms their reasons for changing and makes a commitment to do so (e.g. the person chooses which bus route s/he will take to work, and decides to use it the next day).
- Action: an individual undertakes the desired behaviour (e.g. the person catches the bus).
- Maintenance: the behaviour is sustained and consolidated (e.g. the person found the bus ride convenient and affordable and will repeat the journey regularly).

Alternatively, the individual might relapse into their original state at this point (the bus trip was a one-off and the individual will revert to the car).

Source: Worcester 'Choose How You Move' is based on Prochaska et al, 'Stages of Change Theory' in *Changing for Good* (1994)

4 Break things down:'Segmentation'

As a health practitioner, you may be used to seeing general pamphlets or posters that have been designed to convey a message to the widest possible audience. Social marketing recognizes that, to influence people to change their behaviour, information, services and support need to be tailored so that they are responsive to people's differing needs.

Based on your thorough research, you should be able to identify different population 'segments' fairly easily. These will be distinct sub-groups of people who have similar characteristics (e.g. geographical, social, economic, gender-based, age-based or attitudinal). It doesn't necessarily matter how you segment your target audience – as long as you do! Not only will this allow you to respond to people's particular requirements, it will also enable you to direct your resources most effectively. You may wish to focus on the population segment that is the easiest to reach, the most likely to change or the most in need of your support.

This tailored approach is the next benchmark criterion, 'segmentation'.

Box 8.6
Worcester Choose How You Move: 'Segmentation'

'Choose How You Move' segmented its target audience by dividing people into three categories:

- residents, who were further segmented into groups based on their current travel behaviour and attitudes to enable individualized travel marketing;
- schools;
- employers.

For each of these segments, a different support mix was designed. For instance, school travel plans for schools, individualized travel marketing for residents and workplace support for employers.

5 Know your competition

Competition can be considered in terms of the 'baddies' (e.g. the car manufacturers and advertisers who make it 'sexy' to drive 4x4s) and the 'goodies' (e.g. walk to work schemes, public transport providers or fitness promotion initiatives that collectively compete for your audience's attention). Competition isn't always there to be beaten – strong opportunities for learning and partnership work invariably exist and it makes sense to maximize these, and minimize duplication.

In order to work most effectively in your audience's world, you will need to make yourself familiar with the places and faces and alternative offers that compete for their time and attention. By analysing their environment in this way, you will be implementing the next benchmark criterion: 'competition analysis'.

Box 8.7
Worcester Choose How You Move: 'Competition'

The major source of competition for sustainable travel behaviour is the car. Baseline research showed that 66 per cent of all trips were made by car, but that the majority of car journeys could be realistically replaced:

- 20 per cent by public transport;
- 33 per cent by cycling;
- 12 per cent by walking.

Follow-up research allowed project planners to understand:

- why individuals chose to use the car for specific journeys;
- real or perceived barriers that stopped them from using alternatives (e.g. lack of information; infrequent services; inconvenient routes; lack of skills).

Based on this information, project planners enhanced and publicized the alternative transport service to make it a more competitive product and to lessen the relative appeal of the car.

6 Set clear behavioural goals

As you will know from your own experience, raising people's awareness does not always result in changing their behaviour: you can tell people to get vaccinated, or wash their hands, or attend for screening, but this might have no impact on whether or not they *act*. In a similar way, climate change initiatives that focus solely on awareness-raising are unlikely to result in changed behavioural outcomes.

Social marketing does not bombard people with information and never aims exclusively to change what they think or understand. Instead it aims to create tangible changes in what people *do*. Based on their research, the social marketer will aim to set realistic behavioural goals with the target audience, first measuring a clear baseline before the programme begins and then outlining *who* will do *what* by *when*.

This emphasis on measurable changes in action (not just awareness) is the next benchmark criterion: 'behavioural goals'.

You might want to think about how you would go about measuring baselines and increases for 'use of public transport'.

Box 8.8
Worcester Choose How You Move: 'Behavioural Goals'

Based on 2004 baseline figures, targets were set for each mode of transport:

- decrease single occupancy car use by 20 per cent;
- increase cycling by 100 per cent;
- increase use of public transport by 20 per cent;
- increase walking by 20 per cent.

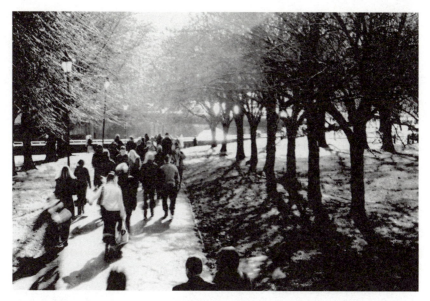

Figure 8.2 On the National Cycle Network, crowded city park path, pedestrians and cyclists make their way towards Bristol Bridge in winter

Source: J Bewley/Sustrans

7 Create an enticing 'offer'

Inevitably, if you ask somebody to adopt a new behaviour, there will be costs involved. These might be monetary (the price of a bus fare or of cycling lessons), but they might also include less tangible costs such as:

- effort (the inconvenience of cycling to work);
- adverse social pressure (being 'the odd one out' in your office);
- embarrassment (feeling silly wearing reflective cycling gear);
- lack of self-belief (not believing you could find your way if you walked to work);
- physical inability (not feeling fit enough to climb the stairs).

Each cost will be immediate and easily identifiable by the target audience.

On the flip side, the behaviours you are promoting will have associated benefits: better health; sense of personal achievement; reduced environmental impact.

Box 8.9
Worcester Choose How You Move: 'Exchange'

Cycling

- **Barriers**: perceived amount of time required; perceived lack of adequate bicycle infrastructure; lack of comfort; car emissions; safety risk; inadequate clothing; generally negative view of cycling as a mode for everyday trips.
- **Incentives**: free bike loan scheme; free cycle lessons; personalized travel plans; personalized route maps; safety advice; improved infrastructure.

Walking

- **Barriers**: as with cycling – time constraints; safety; lack of knowledge about routes.
- **Incentives**: personal travel plans for residents including safety tips; safe routes; lists of routes and journey times for popular local trips; school walking buses; widespread promotion of other benefits, including health and fitness.

Public transport

- **Barriers**: lack of information about services; inconvenience; poor perceptions of potential journey times (over- estimation of the time taken by public transport by nearly two thirds); cost considered too high.
- **Incentives**: tailored information and incentives including timetables about buses visiting the nearest bus stop; free 'taster' tickets; maps of local shopping opportunities; individual advice on how to optimize travel; clear promotion of additional benefits, including environment, congestion, pride in the city, car wear and tear; introduction of new high-frequency bus services and Park & Ride scheme.

However, these benefits will often feel remote and intangible to the target audience.

Your role as a social marketer is to understand what an individual has to give in order to achieve the benefits you are proposing and to minimize these costs as far as possible. This means coming up with an 'offer' that is as easy, convenient and popular as possible to achieve, and introducing a range of benefits, including incentives, recognition and rewards, which are tailored according to specific audiences, based on what they value.

This focus on balancing costs and benefits is the next benchmark criterion: 'exchange'.

8 Design your intervention – mix of methods

Social marketing is different from social advertising or health campaigns because it uses more than just information and avoids relying on a single-pronged approach to behaviour change.

There are four types of intervention that can be combined:

1   Information: let people know what you are asking them to do, why, and what is available to help them.
2   Support: make sure adequate services are in place to allow people to achieve the desired behaviour (e.g. bus services; bike loans; school walking buses).
3   Design: create a physical environment that facilitates the desired behaviour (e.g. bike lanes; outside play spaces; cycle racks).
4   Control: use legislative or fiscal measures to discourage the negative behaviour and encourage the positive (e.g. Congestion Charge Zones; raised parking fees; priority lanes for car sharers).

Your research will guide what's practical in terms of what's actually needed, what might work and what's really possible within your area. If all you're coming up with is an information campaign, it isn't social marketing (even if you develop a broad mix of materials, such as flyers, leaflets, posters and a website).

The use of different types of intervention represents the final benchmark criterion: 'methods mix'.

Box 8.10
Worcester Choose How You Move: 'Methods Mix'

'Choose How You Move' has a strong methods mix, including:

- **Individualized Travel Marketing**: personalized travel information and incentives to try out new ways of getting about including free bus tickets; free bike hire and proficiency training; route maps; home visits from travel experts.
- **Employer Travel Plans**: to encourage alternatives to single-occupancy car commutes, measures such as car-sharing schemes, improved cycling and walking facilities and public transport promotions were used. Flexible-working practices were also encouraged, such as working from home, and tele- or video conferencing.
- **Active School Travel Plans**: schools that create a plan are eligible for a Department for Transport grant for on-site measures to encourage sustainable travel, such as cycle storage, provision of walking buses, lockers and sheltered waiting areas.
- **Infrastructure**: bus shelters, cycle parking, a new walk/cycle bridge over the river, new connecting cycle routes and new bus services.

The benchmark criteria: Summary

Social marketing programmes involve a thorough research and development phase. It is essential not just to jump in feet first and come up with a 'solution', but to invest time in understanding your customer, getting to know the existing situation and pretesting possible options that will respond to people's real life circumstances.

The benchmark criteria provide a checklist of the characteristics of social marketing and will help you to spot any 'gaps' in your programme. Structured project management tools are also very important for the effective design and delivery of interventions. The 'Total Process Planning Model' (TPP) is recommended and is available with supporting tools at www.nsmcentre.org.uk/public/default.aspx?PageID=10. TPP has five steps, which can be summarized as follows:

- Scope: research, hypothesise, understand and research again!
- Develop: build a working blueprint for your programme and pre test it with your audience.
- Implement: put plans into action, and make sure budget and delivery stay on track.
- Evaluate: know what you're measuring, make sure it happens, and continually feed this back into the programme.
- Follow up: don't leave things hanging! If your programme is a one-off, make sure learning gets shared; if it's set to continue, manage it.

By using a social marketing management tool such as this, you will set yourself up to deliver on time and within budget.

Conclusion

Achieving the level of change needed to avoid escalating climate change and improve health at the same time will require pragmatic action from across the health workforce and the wider community – who may not yet recognize the potential for change. By using social marketing techniques you can build a bridge that helps people to make their lives sustainable, by thinking creatively about how best to help individuals, communities and services to achieve the sorts of pro-environmental, pro-health behaviour that will contribute to our overall goal of 'one planet living'. If you do not have the opportunity to undertake a full social marketing programme, you can still use the principles to underpin your daily work. You will also find discussion and examples of community action based on social marketing techniques in Chapter 9.

If this chapter has whetted your appetite, you can consult the English National Social Marketing Centre's case example database at www.nsmcentre.org.uk for a range of social marketing programmes – big and small; local, national and international; from health, environmental and other arenas. Each case example is written up against the benchmark criteria described earlier.

Action points

1   Think about some people whose behaviour you would like to influence: how can you gain insight – get to know them and the world in which they move?
2   What is the tempting 'quick fix' with this group? Why might it backfire? What might be a better long-term solution?
3   What might happen if you just 'tell people what to do'? How can you help them to do it and make it as easy as possible?
4   What can you do that might make your proposal more attractive to your target audience? What or who is competing with you?
5   How can you engage other statutory bodies and stakeholders to secure support for your ideas and pool resources wherever possible?

References

Defra (2004) 'Driving Public Behaviours for Sustainable Lifestyles', available at www.defra.gov.uk/sustainable/government/publications/pdf/desk-research2.pdf

Defra (2008) 'A framework for environmental behaviours', DEFRA, London

DH (2004) 'Choosing health, making healthy choices easier', The Stationery Office, London

DH (2008) 'Ambitions for health', The Stationery Office, London

Glanz, K., Rimer, B.K. and Viswanath, K. (eds) (2002) *Health Behaviour and Health Education: theory, research and practice*, Jossey-Bass, San Francisco

Hastings, G. (2007) *Why Should the Devil Have All The Best Tunes?* Elsevier, Oxford, UK

Kolmuss, A. and Agyeman, J. (2002) 'Mind the gap: why do people act environmentally and what are the barriers to pro-environmental behavior?', *Environmental Education Research*, vol 8, no 3, pp239–260

Prochaska, J.O., Norcross, J.C. and DiClemente, C.C. (1994) *Changing for Good*, William Morrow and Company, New York

9 How to Take Action in the Community

Jenny Griffiths

Our future has the potential to be more rewarding, abundant and enjoyable than today, and by working together we can unleash the collective enthusiasm and genius of our community (that means you!) to make this transition.

Rob Hopkins,
originator of the Transition Town concept
and co-founder of the Transition Network

Summary

Many believe that it is action by communities, rather than by individuals or governments, that is our main hope of creating sustainable communities in the near-enough future to avoid the catastrophic effects of climate change. Localization is the key: a sustainable community has available locally all the essential elements needed to sustain itself and thrive. The international Transition Towns movement has over 120 communities actively pursuing this aim. Chapter 6 described how you can influence important statutory and formal planning processes to contribute to sustainability, whilst this chapter focuses on behaviour change in the community. Community-based social marketing, such as Global Action Plan's EcoTeams, helps people to use group support to change long-standing habits (see Chapter 8 for more information on social marketing). Because many people in high-income societies are not really involved in decisions at group and community level, a lot of time and effort is required to establish trust. But the rewards are very great. Processes to engage the community, empower people to be in control and to create owner-ship, are essential. Successful community change also requires champions with passion and skills to break down personal and organizational barriers: 'No champions, no change.'

Key terms

Carbon neutral: Not adding to the amount of carbon dioxide in the atmosphere, that is, zero carbon emissions.

Champions: People with commitment who want to make a difference by influencing others and breaking down personal and organizational barriers.

Community: An organized system of people in relation to one another.

Discursive social change: A way of tackling entrenched routine and habitual behaviours through social exploration of new alternatives at the group or community level.

Empowerment: A social process that promotes the participation of individuals, organizations and communities in actions with the goal of increased individual and community control, political efficacy, improved quality of life and social justice.

Sustainable community: A community that has available to it locally all the essential elements of life, which is resilient and which lives within its fair share of the Earth's natural resources.

Transition Town: A community in a process of imagining and creating a future that addresses the twin challenges of diminishing energy supplies and climate change and creates the kind of community that we would all want to be part of.

Engaging with communities

What is a community?

Communities have been defined as organized systems of people in relation to one another and the term implies social or emotional ties, a sense of inclusiveness and belonging. Indeed critical to the concept of 'community' for some is the notion of shared consciousness (see Handsley, 2007). A community can be geographical – a cluster of houses, a street or road, a neighbourhood, a village, a town, a school catchment. But many people in the industrialized world, with highly mobile lives, will not feel they have deep social and emotional ties, let alone 'shared consciousness', in the area in which they live and the concept may appear sentimental, which can be a major challenge when engaging with people. Communities based on common characteristics such as ethnicity, age, gender, religion or a shared issue or problem will be easier to identify.

Empowerment

There is a rich literature in the health promotion field concerning strategies and interventions that aim to improve health and address inequalities at a local level, particularly as a result of the growth of community participation and public involvement in the public sector since the 1990s. This learning is relevant to linking health with climate change (for a summary see Lloyd et al, 2007). A number of different concepts and definitions are used, such as 'community action', 'community development', 'community involvement', 'community participation' and 'capacity building' (see Handsley, 2007). (Incidentally, many of these words appear on a list of '100 banned words' that the UK Local Government Association suggests public bodies should not use if they want to communicate effectively. They argue that unless staff talk to residents in a language they understand, people are less likely to get involved in local issues – see www.idea.gov.uk.)

Perhaps the most important of these terms is empowerment, which has been defined as: 'A social process that promotes the participation of individuals, organisations and communities in actions with the goal of increased individual and community control, political efficacy, improved quality of life and social justice.' (Handsley, 2007)

Creating healthy, sustainable, low-carbon communities is likely to require considerably more empowerment – control and actual influence in social, political and economic spheres – than people have currently. Successful community initiatives, for example the Transition Town movement, always empower individuals and communities to gain increased control over the factors that affect their lives, and enhance their sense of well-being and quality of life.

The evidence for community engagement

For community-based health and climate change interventions to be successful, therefore, communities themselves need to be involved. In reviewing the evidence on community engagement, the National Institute for Health and

Clinical Excellence (National Institute for Health and Clinical Excellence, 2008) concluded: 'Approaches that help communities to work as equal partners, or delegate some power to them – or provide them with total control – may lead to more positive health outcomes.'

The National Institute for Health and Clinical Excellence's guidance also recommends that successful initiatives will:

- Take account of existing community activities and area-based initiatives, past experiences and issues raised by the communities involved.
- Understand the gradual, incremental and long-term nature of community engagement activities and ensure mechanisms are in place to evaluate and learn from these processes on a continuing systematic basis.
- Acknowledge the skills and knowledge in the community by encouraging local people to help identify priorities, and contribute to the commissioning, design and delivery of services.
- Identify how power is currently distributed among all those involved, and negotiate and agree with all parties how power will be shared and distributed in relation to decision-making, resource allocation and defining project objectives and outcomes.
- Identify and work with local structures and organizations, offer advice, guidance, mentoring and training if necessary, and empower local people to build partnerships and run community organizations.

It is important to focus on areas of deprivation and to address health inequalities amongst young people, older people, people from black and ethnic minority groups, people with physical health issues, people with mental health issues and people from lower socio-economic groups. All these groups are likely to be particularly affected by the health and social impacts of climate change, because they will live in poorer-quality housing and environments, with more pollution and less resilience to extreme weather events.

Community-based behaviour change

Behaviour is essentially collective; individuals are reluctant to act alone. Our actions are deeply embedded in the wider environment and in the habits, culture and social norms of those around us. If we are to change, we will do so together (Hale, 2008). There is a strong evidence base concerning the social and psychological dimensions of people's behaviour, through mutually supportive groups and networks. Jackson (2005) concluded from his work on motivating sustainable consumption:

> A key lesson from this review is the importance of community-based social change. Individual behaviours are shaped and constrained by social norms and expectations. Negotiating change is best pursued at the level of groups and communities. Social support is particularly vital in breaking habits and in devising new social norms.

Building supportive communities, promoting inclusive societies and encouraging purposeful lives is important to help people break the habits of 'carbon addiction' that have resulted from material goods and services being deeply embedded in the cultural fabric of our lives over the last half century or so.

In Chapter 8, it was noted that habit is a crucial component in a wide variety of environmentally significant activities, for example travel behaviour, shopping patterns, waste disposal (Jackson, 2005). Habits make it easier to cope with day-to-day life, by allowing us to perform routine actions with a minimum of deliberation. They are formed through repetition and reinforcement and – as we all know – are very hard to change.

The social psychologist Kurt Lewin suggested that since many behaviours and practices evolve from social norms and as a result of social expectations, the process of 'unfreezing' existing behaviour patterns needs to take place in a group environment and to involve open and supportive communication. This view is supported by various models within sociology, and resonates with the idea of 'discursive elaboration' that underpins the construction of social identity (Jackson, 2005).

To bring all this theory into real life, the model of discursive social change forms the intellectual basis for Global Action Plan's EcoTeams programme, which has successfully encouraged pro-environmental behaviour changes at the household level through the use of community-based social marketing.

Box 9.1

Case study: Global Action Plan EcoTeams

EcoTeams seek to change people's behaviour at the community level through education, training and support, and give practical advice on how to improve household efficiency, reduce environmental impact and save resources.

The teams comprise six to eight people who each represent their household. With the help of team leaders, they discuss the issues and map out practical actions they can take to reduce their impact in each area. They are encouraged to share their experiences, local knowledge and ideas and to support each other.

Volunteer EcoTeam leaders are recruited and trained by Global Action Plan to recruit and run their own EcoTeams.

The teams consistently achieve changes in energy consumption, waste, water and recycling levels.

Evaluation has shown a 16 per cent average reduction in carbon emissions by participating households.

Source: www.globalactionplan.org.uk/community.aspx

EcoTeams are successful (Global Action Plan, 2008), because:

- The team-based approach provides both support and pressure to change behaviours.
- Household measuring, monitoring and feedback reinforces participants' progress.
- Changes in pre-existing lifestyles become habitual.
- Participation makes people believe that what they do actually makes a difference to the environment, gives them confidence, shows what personal benefits they can get from reducing their environmental impact and, to quote a participant, 'persuaded me that being "green" is normal'.

This and other evidence (see Jackson, 2005) suggests that the careful design of community-based social marketing strategies can have a significant impact on environmental behaviour. Jackson further concludes that the type of social organization that prevails in western high-income societies, that is, individualistic and entrepreneurial, will not be sufficient to achieve the behaviour change demanded by a substantial reduction in carbon emissions and in human ecological impact, required to bring the global ecosystem into balance. Small group and community organization appears to be the best way forward, but is of course a form of social organization that is much less common today in high-income societies than 25 or 50 years ago. It is therefore very important that we get involved in our communities and pool our skills to develop initiatives that bring people together.

Box 9.2

Case study: Action for sustainable living

When a 'green' customer survey was conducted in a Manchester supermarket in 2003, it confirmed that many people are keen to improve their environment, but simply did not have the knowhow. In 2004, with funding from the government, the four people behind the survey launched Action for Sustainable Living, offering practical ways of adopting a more self-sufficient, eco-aware lifestyle – and enabling local people to forge new social links that would strengthen their community.

Action for Sustainable Living is now (2008) funded by the council, businesses and charitable trusts. It employs six paid staff, and 160 volunteers collectively offer 1000 hours of service a month, covering nine categories of work, ranging from fundraising and events to design and IT. A notable project was Old Trafford Action Group's War on Waste campaign, which tackled the problem of mounting litter and engaged an initially unwilling local population in dealing with the mess.

Passers-by are invited to sign a pledge, co-designed with the Stockholm Environmental Institute, to help people reduce their environmental impact and commit to as many eco-steps as they wish. Follow-up revealed that 90 per cent of the 2,400 signatories had kept to some of their eco-pledges and 30 per cent had fulfilled more than their quota.

Source: www.afsl.org.uk

Community-led planning

Community-led planning (see www.communityledplanning.com) is a long-established practice in rural communities in the UK whose use is now being extended into urban settings. With advice and support from an external facilitator, local people take the lead in organizing dialogue with residents, community groups, local institutions and businesses to learn how their community works and to explore solutions to issues that arise. This structured approach can take up to 18 months, making links along the way with relevant statutory bodies and service providers. Very high rates of participation are achieved, with a target of 90 per cent of all households. Hard-to-reach people are enlisted through creative approaches and through the involvement of local groups to which they already belong. The results are grouped into three categories:

1 actions that the community can take itself;
2 actions that need external support to achieve, for example from local government;
3 actions that require external influence over long-term statutory plans (see Chapter 6 for more information).

A nominated community group of new volunteers generated during the plan's development then start to implement the actions that the community can take itself.

Examples of community-based initiatives

Some health practitioners will be involved with health-related community projects as part of their job. Others may be involved in community groups as volunteers. Whether you are active in community projects inside or outside work, you can encourage them to integrate some action on climate change into their activities, perhaps by taking up more active forms of travel, healthier low-carbon diets or reducing the use of gas and electricity. Here are some examples of community-based initiatives on sustainability and climate change to inspire you.

Transition Towns

What we are convinced of is this:

- If we wait for governments, it'll be too little, too late.
- If we act as individuals, it'll be too little.
- But if we act as communities, it might just be enough, just in time. (www.transition.towns.org/)

The international Transition Towns movement is resonating with people keen to play an active part in exploring practical actions that will reduce a community's carbon emissions and improve quality of life and well-being.

Transition Towns aim to organize locally all aspects of life as far as feasible – food, energy, transport, health services and housing. A sustainable community has available locally all the essential elements that it needs to sustain itself and thrive (see Chapter 6). Localization will make the community resilient and able to cope with the potentially damaging effects of climate change. It will also be best placed to achieve the necessary reduction of 1–2 tonnes of carbon per person per year over the next 20 years or so and to substantially reduce its ecological footprint (see Chapter 1). Its citizens will be healthier and it will feel a good place to live.

A Transition Town is 'a community in a process of imagining and creating a future that addresses the twin challenges of diminishing oil and gas supplies and climate change, and creates the kind of community that we would all want to be part of' (www.totnes.transitionnetwork.org). Residents, businesses, public bodies, community organizations and schools are all involved. There are 126 'recognized' Transition Towns, which can be neighbourhoods, districts, villages, towns or cities, in all four UK countries, Ireland, Australia, New Zealand and the USA and a few in Europe. The Transition Towns Network recommends a series of steps towards becoming a Transition Town that include:

- a steering group of four or five individuals to see the project through its initial stages;
- a substantial programme of awareness-raising in the community;
- laying the foundations through extensive networking;
- organizing the 'great unleashing' – a big launch;

- setting up sub-groups for key areas such as food, waste, energy, transport, education;
- developing some visible practical manifestations of the project, such as planting trees;
- facilitating 'the great reskilling' – many of the sustainability skills our grandparents had need to be relearned by current generations, such as repairing, cooking, cycle maintenance, loft insulation, food growing;
- building a bridge to local government.

Transition Towns and health

The links between Transitions Towns and health are many and are well illustrated by food. Totnes, which was the UK's first Transition Town, is linking health promotion and food-growing in people's gardens. The initiative, Totnes Healthy Futures (see www.totnes.transitionnetwork.org) will use a site in central Totnes and is the result of a partnership between Transition Town Totnes, the Totnes Development Trust, the University of Plymouth and Leatside Surgery.

The Totnes Healthy Futures centre aims to help to reduce obesity by promoting exercise, healthy eating and reconnecting people with good, locally grown affordable food. The centre will have a low-carbon building built using mainly local materials, incorporating a public cafe and other spaces. The rest of the site will be dedicated to a model urban food garden, featuring raised beds, soft fruit and medicinal herbs, designed to be an educational resource, showing the potential productivity of urban spaces.

The project is designed to act as a catalyst. Doctors and nurses working in Totnes can see the benefits of encouraging healthier diets and increased exercise. The project will complement the care offered in GP surgeries by providing resources for people with long-term health problems and promoting healthy living to families with young children. Transition Town Totnes also has a garden-share project, a guide to local food, seed and plant swap events, and tree planting, including edible nut trees.

Box 9.3
The health and climate change benefits of trees

Climate change benefits

- Trees act as a carbon dioxide sink, removing carbon dioxide during photosynthesis and releasing oxygen.
- Trees help cool cities, buffering them against heatwaves; urban parks can be up to 5°C cooler than surrounding neighbourhoods.
- The cooling effect reduces power demands during hot weather, which in turn reduces carbon emissions from energy use.

Health benefits

- Having trees near residences and businesses promotes physical activity and improves mental health.
- Trees play a role in reducing air pollution, conserving water, reducing soil erosion and controlling noise.
- Being able to see trees outside a hospital window helps patients to heal faster; a view of trees can also reduce stress in the workplace.
- Trees help to discourage vandalism, graffiti and violence.

Source: Adapted from Frumkin and McMichael (2008)

In England, the Campaign for Greener Healthcare, working with other partners, has launched an initiative to develop a National Health Service Forest of 1.3 million trees planted on and around the NHS estate, contributing to 'The Natural Health Service'. It will link both staff and patients with their local green space. It will be available for commemoration and celebration by patients, relatives and professionals.

Source: www.greenerhealthcare.org

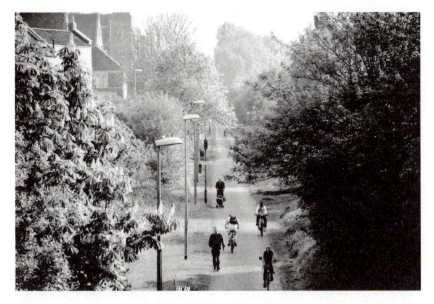

Figure 9.1 Early morning journey to school and commuters on traffic-free greenway through housing area (National Cycle Network)

Source: J. Bewley/Sustrans

The use of Open Space Groups

Many community initiatives, including Transition Towns, use Open Space Groups to involve people. An Open Space event is a gathering in which people discuss issues of heartfelt concern, share ideas, pool their knowledge and create plans for collaborative action. Participants create their own programme of self-managed sessions related to a central theme of strategic importance. There are no invited speakers and just one facilitator to help people to manage the process.

Open Space events help people to work together as equals to decide how they will bring about a mutually desired change for the better and are particularly effective for complex issues. The benefits include:

- people's hearts and minds are fully engaged;
- their heartfelt concerns are surfaced;
- creative and relevant ideas are explored;
- open discussion and collective decision-making are enabled;
- collaboration starts to become the predominant way of working.

An Open Space event follows seven steps: briefing, creating the agenda, sign-up, sessions, session reports, action planning and reflection. (See www.openspaceworld.com/brief_history.htm and www.jackmartinleith.com)

Carbon-neutral communities

Other local initiatives around the world include small communities aiming to become carbon neutral over the next few years. These communities are supporting and inspiring each other using remote communications technology.

In England, the village of Ashton Hayes in Cheshire (population approximately 1000) aims to become the first small community in the country to achieve carbon neutral status: 'We want our children and future generations to know that we tried to do our bit to stem global warming and encourage other communities to follow suit' (Ashton Hayes, 2009). Its inhabitants have reduced their average carbon footprint by 21 per cent in less than two years (2006–2008). Research into the project suggests that 35 per cent of people had become more actively involved in village life and 99 per cent are engaged in environmentally friendly behaviour (Ashton Hayes, 2009).

In Australia, Mount Alexander Sustainability Group is an incorporated not-for-profit organization with 500 members. It aims to protect and enhance the natural and built environments by promoting environmental sustainability within the Mount Alexander Shire, to reduce greenhouse gas emissions by 30 per cent on 2000 levels by 2010 and achieve carbon neutrality by 2015. They say: 'Climate change is the major challenge facing our communities and the natural environment. It is already heating and drying our region' (Mount Alexander Sustainability Group, 2009).

In Canada, the village of Eden Mills has a grass-roots initiative 'to tackle the urgent issue of a warming planet. We want our children and grandchildren to know that we not only cared but tried to do something.' They are aiming to become the first village in North America to achieve carbon neutrality (Eden Mills, 2009).

Carbon Rationing Action Groups

Carbon Rationing Action Groups (or CRAGs) comprise groups of people who have decided to act together to reduce their individual and collective carbon footprints (CRAG, 2009). There are groups in North America and in the UK. They set themselves an annual emissions target or 'carbon ration'. Then they track their emissions over the year by keeping a record of their household energy use and private car and plane travel. At the end of the year, they take responsibility for any 'carbon debt' (emissions over and above their ration) that they have built up. All carbon debts are paid into the group's 'carbon fund' at an agreed rate per kilo of CO_2 debt. The fund is then distributed as agreed by the members of the group.

The aims of the CRAG scheme are:

- to make us all aware of our personal CO_2 footprint;
- to find out if it can help us make radical cuts in our personal CO_2 emissions;
- to help us argue for (or against!) the adoption of similar schemes at a national and/or international level;
- to build up solidarity between a growing community of carbon-conscious people;
- to share practical lower-carbon-living knowledge and experience.

What makes community initiatives successful?

Successful community initiatives give rich reward to those who get involved, mainly because of the social support, sense of belonging and common purpose that is created. Success is usually based on a belief that social relationships are more important than material consumption; a belief that people need communities and that the importance of communities needs to be rediscovered, with all the benefits to well-being that will bring – volunteering is a manifestation of that commitment.

Developing strong relationships in the community

You will have noted that all the examples in the previous section share some common characteristics. They harness the creativity and ingenuity we have used in developing the complex economy and societies of the last 50 years, to build instead a future where the essentials of a fulfilling life are available locally. They develop complex cooperative working relationships at a local level, using networks to connect individuals and families with community groups, schools and businesses.

Billions of words have been written about the importance of engaging local people in local projects. It is not easy. The major obstacles are fear, lack of trust, lack of time and the need for long-term commitment to effect change.

Box 9.4
Case study: Overcoming fear and establishing trust

Bike It: A Sustrans project working directly with children in schools

Nearly half of all children want to cycle to school, but only 2 per cent in the UK do. Why? Because parents are understandably concerned about busy roads and the safety of their children, and schools are often wary of encouraging cycling on health and safety grounds.

> People these days are not used to being involved in decisions that affect them. We need to make it as easy as possible for them to get involved, and stay involved. We particularly need to establish trust with schools and parents, so that they feel able to allow their children to change their travel behaviour. We can only bring about the freedom of children to cycle if we give parents and teachers the peace of mind to let them.

> Without community buy-in our projects would not get off the ground, become accepted by local people or have a lasting impact. We know that practical projects which have had the input of local people are likely to last longer because communities feel a sense of ownership.

Source: Sustrans (2008)

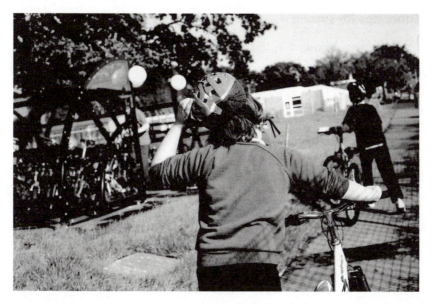

Figure 9.2 A day in the life of Louise Powell, Sustrans Bike It Officer, South Wales. Bike Breakfast at Bryncoch Church in Wales Primary, 2008

Source: J. Bewley/Sustrans

Partnerships

It makes a lot of sense to link your own work with that of other active organizations, such as residents' associations and local government, which will offer access to networks and provide credibility and legitimacy. Most successful community initiatives have developed strong partnerships, which provide a range of support – psychological, financial, access to resources and so on. Many partnerships span the public sector (e.g. local government), local businesses and charitable trusts.

Publicity and information

A well-thought-through communications strategy will make a big difference to the success of your project. Social marketing (see Chapter 8) teaches us to use language and imagery appropriate to the target group. So publicity for young people is likely to be totally different from that appropriate for older people, for example. Be clear about your target group and involve them in devising publicity. Circulate as much information as you can within the limits of your resources.

Other tips for success

The initiatives described in this chapter have some or all of the following features; they:

- are positive about all the benefits to personal and community health and well-being;
- encourage and support people to put their own ideas into practice;
- focus on practical action, such as allotments, switching off appliances, shopping locally, walking or cycling to work, reusing goods;
- connect people with green space and nature and with the sources of their food and energy;
- involve children, who are enthusiastic and take the messages back home, influencing adults' behaviour.

Box 9.5
Case study: Food for life partnership

The Food for Life Partnership is a Big Lottery-funded initiative, led by the Soil Association, to transform food culture in schools and communities across England, bringing together the practical expertise of the Focus on Food Campaign, Garden Organic and the Health Education Trust.

It reaches out through schools to give communities access to seasonal, local and organic food, and to the skills they need to cook and grow fresh food for themselves. They want a new generation to explore how their food choices impact on their health and that of the planet and to rediscover the pleasure of taking time to enjoy real food. Pupils visit farms to see how their food is produced.

All schools in England can enrol with the Food for Life Partnership and work towards Bronze, Silver and Gold Marks for good food culture, rewarding everything from seasonal, local and organic meals, to cooking and growing activity and links with farms. Schools across England are also being selected to become Flagship Schools – exemplars for other schools to learn from.

Source: www.foodforlife.org.uk

No champion, no change!

Finally, champions are essential for successful community initiatives (see Ballard et al, 2007). The presence of a champion – or numerous champions – has consistently proven to be a necessary condition for meaningful change on any scale, in any setting, on any subject, at any time. In addressing climate change, the need for champions is great because of the high stakes and the level of urgency. A champion is someone who combines a number of specific characteristics, of which two 'core qualities' are necessities:

- passion: a personal 'mission' and commitment;
- agency: champions search constantly for ways to maximize their impact on the problem; they actively seek ways to influence others and to break down personal and organizational barriers.

Other qualities often found in champions include:

- cool-headedness, not showing impatience, intolerance and anger, which can lead to isolation due to alienating others, or to burnout;
- courage, tenacity, resilience;
- networking skills;
- a gift for communication and crossing boundaries, understanding participants' own views, translating messages to a wide diversity of audiences.

There are several types of climate change and health champions:

- formal champions: for example elected representatives or senior managers with a formally agreed remit;
- informal visible champions: for whom climate change is part of their primary function in an organization;
- informal, less visible champions: who have a personal interest in the subject.

The champion's role can be isolated and frustrating and helping them to network with other champions can keep them motivated and supported, and develop their performance.

Box 9.6
Case Study: Hinduism and H_2O – Community Champions

London Sustainability Exchange (LSx) was set up in 2001 by a partnership of public, private and voluntary sector organizations to accelerate the transition to a sustainable London. One of their projects, in partnership with the water company Thames Water, is 'Hinduism and H_2O', promoting water efficiency.

The project promotes water conservation with Hindu communities by making the link between scripture and sustainable water consumption. Water symbolizes God's presence, which is why Krishna says, 'I am the taste in water' (Bhagavad Gita 7:8). Programme components include:

- a starter kit of practical water-saving products;
- Hindu temple talks and workshops;
- coffee evening sessions with women's groups;
- a community champions programme which trains trusted figures in the community to run training sessions and provide advice in the home.

The Hinduism and H_2O project has been successful in engaging people, by drawing on the existing communities of faith and place and using community champions. It uses social marketing strategies and techniques, including insight, segmentation and partnership (see Chapter 8).

Source: www.LSx.org.uk

The vision and determination of leaders from outside the established structures of power and wealth has been a driving force behind major social changes in the past, such as gender equality. The prevention of runaway climate change will be no different: community leadership is vital.

Action points

1   What sort of personal life skills would you like to gain to become more self-sufficient and to be able to contribute even more to the community, for example repairing houses and equipment, growing food?

2   Think about what communities you belong to – your road or street, your neighbourhood/village/town – or various interest groups? What is the potential for action on climate change in any of the communities you have identified?

3   What sort of role do you want to play? Are you a champion? An activist in a supporting role? Or willing to help on a pragmatic basis from time to time? Who can you team up with to enable you to do more, in a role you are comfortable with?

4   Do you know people who are champions whom you can link up with? Or how could you set about finding them?

5   This chapter features several case studies. Do you want to join one of these national groups or networks (or their equivalent in other countries), or talk with friends, neighbours or groups about starting something similar in your local area?

6   Think about how you can engage the community, give it a sense of ownership, generate trust, reduce people's fear and help them to be empowered.

7   What partnerships can you create or access to give you support and help you to network with others?

8   Brief yourself further and try out Open Space Technology as a way of involving a community of people in developing a plan for change.

References

Ashton Hayes (2009) available at http://goingcarbonneutral.co.uk (accessed 14 February 2009)

Ballard, S., Weston, R. and Black, D. (2007) *Guidance: champions for change*, ESPACE – Planning in a changing climate, available at www.espace-project.org/part1/publications.pdf39.pdf (accessed 9 January 2009)

CRAGs (2009) Carbon Rationing Action Groups, available at www.carbonrationing.org.uk (accessed 14 February 2009)

Eden Mills (2009) available at www.goingcarbonneutral.ca (accessed 14 February 2009)

Handsley, S. (2007) 'The potential for promoting public health at a local level: Community strategies and health improvement', in Lloyd, C.E., Handsley, S., Douglas, J., Earle, S. and Spurr, S. (eds) *Policy and Practice In Promoting Public Health*, Sage Publications, London (in association with the Open University)

Frumkin, H. and McMichael, A. J. (2008) 'Climate change and public health: thinking, communicating, acting', *American Journal of Preventive Medicine*, vol 35, pp403–410

Global Action Plan (2008) 'An Introduction to EcoTeams', available at www.globalactionplan.org.uk/community.aspx (accessed 10 June 2009)

Hale, S. (2008) *The New Politics of Climate Change: why we are failing and how we will succeed*, Green Alliance, London

Hopkins, R. (2008) *The Transition Handbook: from oil dependency to local resilience*, Green Books, Totnes, Devon

Lloyd, C.E., Handsley, S., Douglas, J., Earle, S. and Spurr, S. (eds) (2007) *Policy and Practice in Promoting Public Health*, Sage Publications, London (in association with the Open University) (see in particular Part II *Promoting public health at a local level*)

Jackson, T. (2005) 'Motivating Sustainable Consumption: A Review of Evidence on Consumer Behaviour and Behavioural Change', a report to the Sustainable Development Research Network, www.sd-research.org.uk/post.php?p=126 (accessed 9 January 2009)

Mount Alexander Sustainability Group (2009) available at http://masg.org.au (accessed 14 February 2009)

National Institute for Health and Clinical Excellence (2008) 'Community Engagement', NICE public health guidance 9, NICE, London

Sustrans (2008) 'Are we learning to love community involvement? *The Network*, Issue 9, Winter 2008, pp10–11, Sustrans, Bristol

10 How to Help Organizations to Take Action

Jenny Griffiths and Lucy Reynolds

Never doubt that a small group of thoughtful committed citizens can change the world; indeed, it is the only thing that ever has.

Margaret Mead

Summary

It is finally being recognized that the global economy is well on the way to destroying its own ecological base. Companies large and small are reducing their own emissions, greening their supply chains and beginning to encourage customers in environmental behaviours, partly in the interests of their own long-term survival. But more action needs to be taken quickly. The workplace is a vital setting for change because many of us spend much of our lives at work and it has the potential to be a mainspring of collective action. Workplace health promotion programmes are intrinsically valuable and can lead to increased business benefits, including reduced sickness absence, improved productivity and customer loyalty. They can also be integrated synergistically with action to reduce carbon emissions. For example, promotion of exercise through walking or cycling to work will both improve health and reduce car usage. Health practitioners and health organizations are uniquely well placed, both to instigate integrated workplace health and climate change activity in their own workplaces and also to encourage change in partner organizations, community organizations and small and medium sized enterprises. The key elements of successful organizational strategies are described, including the importance of board leadership.

Key terms

Corporate social responsibility: Positive management of the environmental and social impact of a business.

Supply chain: All activities from primary suppliers through to the point of sale/delivery, often involving a number of companies.

SMEs: Small and medium sized enterprises. In the UK, 99 per cent of businesses are SMEs of under 250 employees. They employ 14 million people and account for 50 per cent of UK turnover.

Tailoring: Interventions that are tailored to specific audience segments rather than relying on 'blanket' approaches.

The workplace as a setting for change

The aim of this chapter is to suggest that it would be worth your spending a little of your time engaging with either the organization in which you work and/or another organization in your area, to stimulate some action on reducing greenhouse gas emissions and improving health. There are three main reasons for this suggestion:

- Over half the UK population spend an estimated 60 per cent of their waking lives at work (Bull et al, 2008). The workplace offers unique opportunities to engage citizens in health-promoting behaviour that is also environmentally beneficial, and to change the way organizations are run to make it easier for people to alter their behaviour.
- Workplaces offer opportunities for promoting communal effort, developing social networks, identifying and developing opinion leaders and champions, to create collective action.
- Finally, business plays an important role in championing national and local government action to tackle climate change, so partnerships with the corporate sector can add considerable muscle to your efforts.

Box 10.1
The °Climate Group

- Launched in 2004 to help speed up the shift to a low-carbon economy.
- Has over 50 corporate and government members from companies, states and regions around the world.
- Believes reducing emissions is good for business.
- 'Breaking the Climate Deadlock' – a major initiative to help build high-level political and business support in key countries for a new and ambitious international climate change agreement post-2012.
- Aims to create 'game-changing' initiatives – projects that will make the biggest difference in the least amount of time.
- Headquarters is in the UK, with offices in the USA, Australia, China and Hong Kong.

Source: www.theclimategroup.org

As a health practitioner, there are four types of organization that you might want to influence to help to reduce their carbon emissions and promote the health of their workforce and the wider community, either as part of your work or on a voluntary basis in the community:

1   the health service;
2   local government;
3   a large organization, such as a supermarket chain;
4   a local small or medium sized business or non-governmental organization.

If you work in public health or health care, Chapter 11 gives ideas and information on how your organization can make a major contribution to reducing carbon emissions and promoting health at the same time. This chapter is about influencing all the other organizations in which people work or with which we interact in our daily lives – partner organizations, suppliers, in the community, when shopping, or obtaining services. We come into contact with organizations through work, though leisure and as citizens in a local community, for example residents' associations.

This chapter offers you some ideas and guidance, most of which is relevant to all organizations. The final sections offer specific insights on different types of organization and on the key areas of travel planning, food and energy efficiency.

There are two main drivers for action – corporate social responsibility and workplace health – both of which have benefits for commercial and non-commercial organizations financially and in enhancing their reputation to attract more customers. The profit margin will naturally be a primary motivator for the corporate sector, so the trick is to present opportunities for health promotion and carbon reduction in ways that show how they can enhance profitability.

Towards a sustainable commercial sector

The global business community has until relatively recently opposed action on climate change, particularly through the Global Climate Change Coalition (Hale, 2008). Today climate change is 'dramatically rewriting the rules for business, investors and consumers' (Worldwatch Institute, 2008). The commercial sector now overwhelmingly accepts the science and urgency of climate change. The first tentative steps are being taken to create the world's first ever 'sustainable' global economy. A whole range of major companies have announced environmental initiatives since about 2005, from McKinsey & Company to Wal-Mart and Tesco. In America, 27 major corporations, including household names like Xerox, have been actively urging the US Congress to pass legislation regulating greenhouse gas emissions, which would have been unthinkable just a few years ago (Worldwatch Institute, 2008).

This shows the gradual growth of understanding of the importance of wider measures of economic well-being (see Porritt, 2007), for example the Index for Sustainable Economic Welfare, which measures social and environmental activity and impacts, not only growth in production of goods and services.

However, businesses respond above all to market signals. Further shifts in public attitudes are needed to create new market pressures and opportunities for corporate action – which is where your role as a health practitioner comes in.

Corporate social responsibility (CSR)

CSR – or simply corporate responsibility – has been around for several decades and can be seen simply as good corporate governance. It can be received with cynicism, but is delivering real results in implementing environmental and community strategies, with a knock-on effect on customer and staff behaviour patterns. CSR is closely related to sustainable development (see Chapter 3) and can deliver tangible environmental and social benefits along with financial savings and benefits in maintaining or growing customer market share.

The business case for CSR is that a company that is positively managing its environmental and social impact is more efficient, and better at coping with challenges and best placed to outperform others in difficult economic times (Business in the Community, 2008). The evidence base for improved company performance is international. CSR strengthens public trust and therefore sustains the value attributed by customers to the company's products – it enhances customer loyalty. It reflects the growing expectations that society globally is placing on business to behave responsibly. CSR is generally seen to have several strands:

- Developing the organization's workforce, including managing the health and well-being of staff to help increase productivity.
- Trading responsibly and ethically, including responsible supply chain management.
- Protecting the environment, including reducing carbon emissions.
- Working in partnership with communities.

CSR is a valuable 'hook' for health practitioners to use for both initial communication and subsequent activities on health and climate change in business settings.

Business engagement with climate change

In the business community, climate change is now seen as the greatest challenge facing society today. Environmental issues are placed at the top of the list of concerns likely to gain the most public and political attention over the next few years (Corporate Citizenship, 2008).

One of the major reasons for the commercial sector embracing carbon reduction has been research concluding that the damage from global climate change could equal as much as 8 per cent of global economic output by the end of this century. According to the World Bank, some 39 countries could expect a decline of 5 per cent or more in wealth when accounting measures also include environmental losses, such as unsustainable forest harvesting and depletion of non-renewable resources. For ten countries, the decline ranged from 25 to 60 per cent (Worldwatch Institute, 2008). In other words, it is finally being recognized that the global economy is now destroying its own ecological base.

As Sir Terry Leahy, Tesco chief executive has put it:

> **For every £1 we spend now on tackling climate change, we are saving our children anywhere between £5 and £20 at today's value. Failure to act means risking economic and social disruption on the scale of the great wars and economic depression of the last century. (Leahy, 2008).**

He could easily have added damage to health.

The Confederation of British Industry (CBI) published a report in 2007 on what British firms can do to fight global warming (CBI, 2007). The report was written by 18 chairmen and chief executives of firms including British Airways, Tesco, BT, Shell and Ford. The position of business has changed radically over the last five years from one of instinctive opposition to environmental regulation and taxation, to a view that businesses need to be 'green to grow'. This is partly because tackling climate change is now seen as a major economic opportunity and a growing recognition that failure to act now will mean that the costs of tackling climate change in the future will be much higher. Although the business community still speaks with forked tongues as it continues to lobby for new airports and roads.

There are four main short-term arguments you can use in communicating with business, in addition to the 'big picture' summarized above:

- Realizing bottom-line efficiency savings: 'Common sense is not always common practice'. There are often opportunities to reduce waste in procurement, fuel use, travel and waste management that can save money.

- Winning new business: increasingly procurers are looking to green their supply chains, which means a company needs to demonstrate its green credentials in order to win business.
- Building reputation with stakeholders: clients, partners and staff increasingly want to see the environment being taken seriously and reduce risks by working with a responsible and forward-thinking business.
- Innovating change: there are increasing opportunities in the marketplace for new products and services that take the environment into consideration.

Workplace health programmes and climate change

So you should find the door at least ajar when you engage in conversation on climate change and health with an organization. But most organizations could do much, much more and the seriousness of climate change means that further action is needed quickly. Health practitioners have a strong argument to encourage more commitment by citing the additional health benefits (see Chapter 4).

Health practitioners can play a hugely important role in supporting work-based change through integrating workplace health and climate change programmes. Most experience exists with workplace health programmes. For example in England Well@Work, led by the British Heart Foundation and funded by the Department of Health, Sport England and the Big Lottery Fund, has reached up to 10,000 employees in 32 workplaces across England over two years. The evaluation, undertaken by Loughborough University (Bull et al, 2008) shows that workplace health programmes can have an impact on levels of physical activity, fruit and vegetable intake, staff morale, communications and working atmosphere. It should be comparatively straightforward to extend such programmes to take on board the reduction of carbon emissions. For example, people taking part in active travel schemes in the Well@Work programme spent an extra 24 minutes on average walking or cycling to and from work.

Workplace health programmes are demonstrably effective, for example in encouraging employees to be more physically active (National Institute for

Health and Clinical Excellence, 2008). What we need now are programmes that integrate health promotion in the workplace with low-carbon living and working practices in the key areas of reducing car dependence, better food and reduced consumption of energy. Exciting opportunities exist to create cross-cutting interventions:

- Walking/cycling to work: exercise that costs nothing and benefits the environment.
- Using the stairs: save energy and burn calories.
- Food policy at work: sourced locally, organic where possible (which is environmentally protective), more fruit and vegetables, which are lower in carbon and healthier, and less meat consumption and processed food.

Very few such integrated health and climate change programmes yet exist – but the potential is there for you to seize!

Benefits of workplace health promotion to employers and employees

One of the many challenges facing public and private sector employers alike is the rising cost of ill health. In the fiscal year 2005–2006, an estimated 30.5 million working days were lost as a result of work-related illnesses and injuries in England. On average, each sick person took 16 days off work in that 12-month period (National Institute for Health and Clinical Excellence, 2008). Investing in the health of employees can bring business benefits such as reduced sickness absence, improved productivity, increased loyalty, better staff retention and reduced costs for employers.

Employers can introduce programmes to improve health and well-being at work, which will increase employee satisfaction with the work environment and encourage healthy attitudes to diet, exercise, smoking and stress.

In the UK, only 3 per cent of employers offer a comprehensive provision of occupational health and related support services (TUC, 2007). Whilst companies recognize the bottom-line benefits of a healthy workforce, developing and implementing a strategy is a challenge for them – particularly linking health promotion with climate change. This is where health practitioners, especially public health and health promotion specialists, can help. Health organizations, especially commissioners, should act as a central source of good practice on workplace health and climate change.

Box 10.2

Case Study: Business Health Network, Plymouth

The Business Health Network was set up in 1995 to work directly with employers and organizations in and around Plymouth. It offers:

- Recognition of an employer's commitment to health and well-being at work through the Health@Work awards.
- Practical help and support to implement policies and initiatives at work to improve health and well-being in the workplace.
- Information about other organizations and policies to support the work of an employer.
- Information about local health services to inform employees and their families.

The Business Health Network is part of NHS Plymouth's Public Health Development Unit (PHDU). The PHDU is responsible for protecting and promoting the health of everyone living and working in Plymouth, including the prevention of major diseases and conditions including mental health issues, coronary heart disease, cancers and strokes.

The purpose of the Health@Work awards is to help workplaces implement healthy living policies, by recognising businesses that demonstrate a commitment to employees' health.

Awards are tailored to each workplace's level of practice, using a points system.

The Health@Work awards come under a number of categories that could easily be extended to include low-carbon lifestyles, including healthy eating and physical activity.

Source: www.plymouthpct.nhs.uk/healthandwellbeing/Pages/businesshealthnetwork.aspx

You can make a difference

Successful change in organizations requires leadership, appropriate attitudes, knowledge, culture, skills and competencies, tools and resources. Do not underestimate your own impact on an organization, even if you have very little time. There is evidence that employees have a particularly significant role in pressing for change, so linking up with one or two of them, in an organization that you approach, is a good starting point (Corporate Citizenship, 2008). Tim Smit, chief executive and co-founder of the Eden Project in Cornwall, is a great believer in the Tinkerbell Theory – from Peter Pan, where Tinkerbell drinks some poison and Peter turns to the audience for help and asks them to clap their hands if they believe Tinkerbell can be saved. Smit says if you get three or four people to believe in something, they will each convince three or four others and they will in turn persuade others... This is how change happens in daily life.

Eleven key steps for organizational strategies

Effective organizational strategies for health and climate change, be they for your household, for a small group, a team, a department or a large organization, will have the following 11 key steps in them somewhere (though change does not in practice happen in such an orderly manner!). The examples below link reducing carbon dioxide emissions (through less car usage) with increasing physical activity. Exercise initiatives may be relatively simple to 'market' to employees as they are fun and easy to link in with social events (Bull et al, 2008) and therefore a good place to start.

Box 10.3
The benefits of walking to work

- There is a significant link between commuting to work by car and being overweight or obese.
- But just 90 minutes of exercise each week can cut the number of sick days employees take by half.
- Employees who take part in exercise initiatives run by their workplace report that they enjoy their work more, have increased concentration and mental alertness and better rapport with colleagues.
- If fewer employees travel by car, you'll be lowering your carbon footprint.
- You could save on parking costs too.
- Add information on walking to your intranet, bulletins and staff newsletters.
- Offer people walking route maps that show stations and landmarks within walking distance of your place of work. Include these in information packs and on websites to encourage suppliers, potential new employees and visitors to walk to your office.
- Produce specific walking routes for individual members of staff.
- Start a buddy system for colleagues who live close to each other to walk to and from work together.
- Ask your Chief Executive Officer and/or Chairman to make walking part of his/her journey.

Source: www.walkingworks.org.uk

---

1 Calculate or estimate your carbon footprint and collect or estimate data on health, for example physical activity levels

You can find a carbon footprint for your local authority area in England on the internet, published by Defra – search for 'emissions of carbon dioxide for local authority areas'. (Note that this gives the UK national average as 7.9 tonnes per capita, which is lower than that quoted elsewhere in this book, because the data excludes the following greenhouse gas emissions: from the production of goods that are imported, from industry in the EU Emissions Trading

Scheme, from refineries, power stations, shipping and aviation.) But it is a useful comparative set of data.

For data on health in England, go to your local Public Health Observatory website. You can make estimates initially. For example 65 per cent of men and 76 per cent of women aged over 16 are not physically active enough to meet the national recommendations of spending 30 minutes on five or more days a week involved in at least moderately intense activities (National Institute for Health and Clinical Excellence, 2008).

2 Set carbon reduction and health targets

The English national carbon reduction target is 80 per cent by 2050, which equates to 4 per cent each year. The English Government's Climate Change Committee is urging us to cut emissions by 30 per cent between 2005 and 2020. But it is much more motivating to set short-term targets, such as 5 per cent in the next year, or 20 per cent over five years. We really do need to make significant progress quickly.

For physical activity, you could aim over the next year to have over half the workforce spending more than 30 minutes on five or more days a week involved in moderate exercise.

3 Talk about a vision of a better, healthier, low-carbon future

See Chapter 6, to help people see all the positive benefits. Quality of life through relationships and nature will be the new status symbol. Everything will be more local – shopping, business networks, amenities. People will spend much more time in their local community and waste much less time travelling.

4 Choose specific actions

Choose actions that will both reduce carbon emissions and promote health, such as active travel and reducing car use, or improving diets by eating less meat and processed foods and wasting less food.

5 Involve everyone

Maximize the opportunity for all employees and managers to participate. Ensure that programmes are based on consultation with staff and that they are

Box 10.4
Carbon Clubs

A Carbon Club is a group of like-minded people who want to tackle environmental and climate change issues to reduce their carbon footprint and protect the environment.

BT launched them in 2007 in response to feedback from employees and now has more than 120 Carbon Clubs around the world.

Source: www.btplc.com/climatechange

involved in planning and design, as well as monitoring activities on an ongoing basis. Identify and train champions who will encourage their colleagues to get moving and help monitor action in the office.

6 Communicate

Use a wide variety of methods: posters and signage, flyers and leaflets, newsletters and e-bulletins, providing information about the benefits of making healthier, low-carbon choices. More creative messaging techniques include drama, song and video. Signposting to existing projects and activities within the workplace and locally in the community and promotion of local and national events can also be helpful. Opportunities for social networking electronically and in person generate energy and commitment.

Successful behaviour change results from bringing people together, focusing on positive change, simple presentation and communication that is fun, engaging, imaginative and interactive. For example, the environmental organization Global Action Plan (www.globalactionplan.org.uk) has five toolkits designed to involve employees in practical environmental action, quickly, cost-effectively and with minimum disruption, with the catchy titles of: Hot Air; Carbon Detectives; Eco-driving Simulator; Watch your Waste; The Paper Trail.

7 Programmes and services to develop skills and reward achievement

Ideas include information sessions about healthy, low-carbon choices (for example about food), workplace activity challenges, lunchtime led walks, participation in charity events, workplace teams entering into local competitions or award schemes, certificates for individuals or groups recognizing their achievements.

The involvement of 'VIPs' from the local community can give positive feedback and recognition. Hands-on activities such as carrying out waste audits and trials of growing food are also effective. It needs to be exciting!

8 Supportive work environment

Such things as the provision of bike racks, changing facilities and showers, improvements to the lighting and decoration of stairwells and changes to canteen menus, create supportive physical and cultural environments that strengthen and enhance healthy practices.

9 Workplace policies

Policies are needed to make healthy, low-carbon choices easier, such as home working, flexitime, travel plans, a workplace food policy.

10 Shout about it!

Tell people about the great things you're doing and how they can join in.

11 Measure your impact

Measure your impact on employees' carbon emissions and health, even if indirectly, and monitor progress qualitatively as well by seeking feedback from staff, managers and other partners. Continuously review how you are doing.

Role of boards and senior management

The engagement of chief executives and boards of directors, or trustees, or the council executive, is crucial. A non-executive champion can be particularly helpful. In all sectors, the board is there to oversee the organization's policies and to ensure they are implemented. The board therefore has the authority to ensure that sustainable, health-promoting policies become part of an organization's core commitment. In the long term, programmes must be supported by management and have dedicated resources.

Box 10.5
Building sustainability into leadership: Seven competences

- thinking about the big picture of the interconnections between health and climate change;
- anticipating radical change;
- articulating health services that thrive in a low-carbon world;
- inspiring change – a 'can do' culture;
- connecting carbon reducing actions with the business;
- working collaboratively and in partnerships;
- walking the talk – leading by example through personal behaviour.

Source: Dr Chris Tuppen, BT's Director of Sustainable Development, presentation at the launch of NHS Carbon Reduction Strategy, London, 27 January 2009 (see www.sdu.nhs.uk)

The importance of partnerships

Partnership working can enhance the effectiveness of programmes, share knowledge and resources and allow the widest possible audience to be reached. It can also help to tie together activities that promote health and protect the environment.

For example, the Walking Works scheme (see Box 10.3) is endorsed by a range of partners from a variety of sectors, including: Sustrans, London Sustainability Exchange, Streets Alive, Asthma UK, Walk England, Act Travel Wise, Walk BUDi, the Civic Trust, National Heart Forum and Walking the Way to Health. Walking Works has also recruited a range of organizations across the country to be campaign partners to try out methods and tactics to see what works – and what does not. The participating organizations benefit both directly from their involvement and from raising their profiles and the Walking Works scheme ensures that their programmes are fully tested and appropriately marketed.

Another example is the endorsement by the internationally prestigious United Nations Environment Programme (UNEP) of the campaign Appetite for Action, launched by Sky's partnership with Global Action Plan, an interactive programme aimed at primary schools across the UK and Ireland, which provides a framework for teaching and learning about sustainable food (www.appetite-foraction.org.uk).

Organizations large and small...

Small and medium sized enterprises (SMEs)

SMEs make up most businesses. They are numerous in wholesale, retail, financial and business services, real estate, construction, hotels, restaurants etc. With a relatively small turnover and few staff, they can be focused on business survival and do not always have time for wider agendas. By befriending an SME, you may therefore make a real difference and there will be many within easy reach of you. Take time to understand them and their needs and offer targeted, tailored support. You will need to develop a long-term relationship and take one step at a time, because both you and the organization will have limited time. Many SMEs will not have training budgets and find external training courses too broad in scope.

Lacking substantial corporate management resources, SMEs may welcome practical help with both workplace health and carbon reduction. They will want one-to-one reviews, advice and practical proposals, for example on travel and exercise. You may also be able to assist them with greening their supply chain. Help them to promote their achievements and raise their public profile, which will in turn generate more business for them.

Box 10.6

Case Study: Focus Consultants (UK) Ltd

Focus Consultants (UK) Ltd, a Nottingham SME, adopted a travel plan as an integral part of its business planning. The company's growth required it to move to a new head office one mile north of Nottingham city centre. The new location increased employees' reliance on the car and this was seen to be incompatible with the company's corporate objectives. A business travel plan was developed, which provided facilities for home and tele-working, and supported alternative travel options.

Focus was able to cut business travel costs by over £7000 per year, achieve an 11 per cent shift from single car occupancy to more sustainable modes of transport and a 9 per cent reduction in business miles, and gained a happier and more productive workforce. Infrastructure provisions included:

- desktop computers to enable staff to work from home;
- laptop computers and portable printers for consultants, allowing them to work between appointments without needing to return to the office;
- configuration of the central computer server to permit remote access;
- focus on encouraging staff to car share on business and commuter journeys by highlighting the benefits and giving guarantees of a ride home;
- a new computer aided design plotter for technical drawings removed the need to travel to the local reprographics company.

Source: www.energysavingtrust.org.uk/business/Global-Data/Publications/TE229-Case-Study-Focus-Consultants-Travel-plan-supports-growth-strategy-for-SME

Large companies

This example illustrates the point made at the beginning of the chapter: that companies are realizing that it is in their interests to take climate change seriously.

Box 10.7
Case study: EDF Energy

EDF Energy has committed to reduce the carbon footprint from its own use of energy by 30 per cent by 2012 and is extending its impact through projects to help its customers reduce their energy use.

EDF Energy generates, distributes and supplies electricity and gas. The company has committed to transform itself into a sustainable business. EDF Energy's 'Our Climate Commitments' set a target to reduce the carbon intensity of the company's electricity generation by 60 per cent by 2020.

EDF Energy recognized that before it could encourage customers and employees to reduce carbon emissions, it would need to put its own house in order. It has cut emissions from offices and depots, reduced the volume of materials sent to landfill and is making its existing power stations more efficient. The company is also investing in new renewable energy technologies including wind and marine power.

The company has developed an energy efficiency toolkit for business customers, which helps them reduce energy use through a five-step process. It has given tailored support, for example evaluating three of Royal Mail's sites, identifying energy saving potential of up to 43 per cent.

For its retail customers, EDF Energy has introduced the 'Read, Reduce and Reward' scheme which rewards customers for reducing their energy consumption. Over 300,000 retail customers had signed up to the scheme by 2008.

EDF Energy believes these initiatives will attract new customers, increase staff satisfaction and maintain the support of other stakeholders.

Evaluation of impacts:

- Company carbon footprint reduced by 19 per cent by 2008.
- Office operations' energy costs reduced by £310,000 a year.
- The Energy Efficiency Toolkit brought in over £30m of new revenue.
- Over 1000 businesses have implemented the toolkit with an average energy saving of 10 per cent.

Source: Business in the Community Environmental Impact Awards, www.bitc.org.uk/awards_for_excellence/awards_for_excellence_winners/big_tick_2008.html#environmental_impact_awards)

Local authorities

'Climate change is the most important long-term priority for local government. It is a test of the sector's credibility and reputation. It is as important now as public health and sanitation were to our Victorian predecessors.' (Sir Simon Milton, Chair of the UK Local Government Association – see www.lga.gov.uk).

Sustainable development is now at the heart of the performance framework for local authorities in the UK. The government's statutory guidance emphasizes that sustainability should be central to the content of the two key local plans, the Local Strategic Partnership's Sustainable Community Strategy and its Local Area Agreement. You will find information in Chapter 6 about how to work with local authorities on planning to help to create healthier, sustainable, low-carbon communities.

The purpose of this note here is simply to remind you that local authorities are themselves large organizations with workforces who can be mobilized for healthy, low-carbon living, and therefore benefit from the workplace strategies described earlier.

Sustainable travel plans

A sustainable travel plan aims to reduce car use (and therefore carbon emissions) by promoting and supporting all the possible alternatives.

A well-designed travel plan can save organizations money, significantly reduce car use and promote physical activity (and therefore health and well-being) (Faculty of Public Health, 2009). Every organization should have one!

The three key areas for action (Department for Transport, 2008) are:

- Promoting 'active travel' such as cycling and walking to and from work and to meetings (including visitors and patients where appropriate), using public transport rather than the car, 'guaranteed ride home' schemes (such as emergency taxis for staff who car share or use public transport); reimbursing cycle mileage.
- Reducing the need to travel, for example by homeworking, increased use of teleconferencing and videoconferencing rather than physical meetings.
- Incentives to share cars and drive smaller, more fuel-efficient cars including reducing single occupancy through promoting car share schemes and car pool schemes.

'We call it self-powered commuting!' – Anthony House, Google Office, London

---

Box 10.8
Case Study: Cyclescheme

Cyclescheme is the UK's number one provider of tax-free bikes for the government's Cycle to Work initiative. Employees make big savings on new bikes, employers get a healthier workforce and save money!

Cyclescheme helps employers of all sizes to set up and run successful Cycle to Work schemes, working with a supplier network of over 1,000 independent bike shops.

The scheme is run in strict accordance with the government's green travel plan. Cyclescheme provides hire agreements for employees and a free secure website for voucher processing.

Source: www.cyclescheme.co.uk/

Figure 10.1 Walking and cycling directional sign on National Cycle Network, Route 4, Castle Park, Bristol

Source: J. Bewley/Sustrans

Sustainable events

To protect our natural resources, it is important that events (meetings, conferences, courses) are as sustainable as possible. Think about the following when planning an event:

- Encourage participation through teleconferencing and videoconferencing rather than personal travel, where appropriate and feasible; it takes practice, but saves a lot of carbon and time travelling.
- The choice of venue – is it easily accessible by public transport? Are hotels within walking distance of the venue?
- Offer a shuttle bus or van from train stations to the venue; provide maps for walking and public transport information to the venue.
- Delegate packs and giveaways – avoid bags (even if they are not plastic) as they will probably not be used again. Minimize the amount of paper – the UK Faculty of Public Health makes most of its conference-related information available only electronically.

- Provide tap water, not bottled water.
- Catering – reduce food miles by sourcing food locally, with as much healthy fruit and vegetables as possible. Minimize meat and processed food. The catering at the UK Public Health Association's 2009 Annual Forum was entirely vegetarian, following consultation with delegates at the previous year's forum.
- Provide reusable mugs at the beginning of the event, use reusable dishes and glassware. Provide teaspoons, bulk sugar and milk in jugs.
- Avoid excess heating.
- Include the three Rs – reduce, reuse, recycle – in contracts with suppliers.
- Ensure recycling bins are numerous, conveniently located and well marked.
- Make all participants, sponsors and hosts aware of your policies and how you have implemented them.
- After the event, evaluate how it went and make plans for improvements.

Energy efficiency

There are of course many ways to reduce energy consumption in the workplace:

- homeworking where appropriate and feasible;
- use of videoconferencing instead of travelling to meetings;
- reducing overseas travel;
- turning lights and equipment off when not needed, turning heating down.

You could remind your contacts in organizations that there is growing pressure to report publicly on energy efficiency. For example, in Britain the government's Carbon Reduction Commitment is due to be rolled out from 2010. This will require businesses to purchase carbon credits for the energy that they use. Bonuses will be awarded for good performance, with penalties for those who fail to reduce their energy. Organizations will be ranked on their performance to provide an extra incentive for businesses who want to show their green credentials.

Action points

1   Are there opportunities in your working life to bring together health promotion and reducing carbon emissions, for example through using the car less and walking or cycling to work?

2   Can you see any opportunities for achieving real change quickly in workplaces you know or can get to know, and how would you 'sell' those opportunities?

3   Why are physical activity and food good areas for 'win–wins' on both reducing carbon emissions and promoting health?

4   How do you think change happens (Tim Smit, who founded the Eden Project, says that if you get three or four people to believe in something, they will each convince three or four others and so on)?

5   Successful workplace projects will have some ongoing measurement of progress, so what specific goals and targets do you want to set? For reducing carbon emissions, set short-term goals such as 5 per cent less over the next year.

6   It's not just about 'telling people what to do' – what mix of methods do successful interventions require? Think about project control, education, design, support etc.

7   How can you involve people in the design of programmes? How can you communicate what you want to happen in a fun, engaging and imaginative way?

8   Can you make your meetings, events, conferences more sustainable? It's another area where you can have a quick impact and enhance your organization's reputation.

9   Have you any opportunities to influence chairs, chief executives and directors to exercise leadership and see quick benefits?

10 Are you and your organization shouting about what you have achieved? Tell your patients, clients, customers, local and national elected officials...

References

Bull, F.C., Adams, E.J., Hooper, P.L. and Jones, C.A. (2008) 'Well@Work: A Summary Report and Calls to Action', British Heart Foundation, London

Business in the Community (2008) 'Corporate Responsibility and the Financial Crisis: Business in the Community's Response', available at www.bitc.org.uk (accessed 4 January 2009)

CBI (2007) Climate Change: everyone's business, CBI, London

Corporate Citizenship (2008) 'The Shape of Corporate Citizenship in 2008', available at www.corporate-citizenship.com (accessed 4 January 2009)

Department for Transport (2008) 'The Essential Guide to Travel Planning', available at www.dft.gov.uk/pgr/sustainable/travelplans/work/ (accessed 10 June 2009)

Faculty of Public Health (2009) Sustaining a Healthy Future: taking action on climate change, 2nd edition, Faculty of Public Health, London

Hale, S. (2008) The New Politics of Climate Change: why we are failing and how we will succeed, The Green Alliance, London

Leahy, T. (2008) 'We must go green', The Guardian, 3 September, p9

Marches Energy Agency (2008) 'Low Carbon Leadership – A workbook for decision makers', Marches Energy Agency in partnership with Energy Saving Trust

National Institute for Health and Clinical Excellence (2008) 'Workplace health promotion: how to encourage employees to be physically active', NICE public health guidance 13, NICE, London, available at www.nice.org.uk

Porritt, J. (2007) Capitalism As If the World Matters, Earthscan, London

TUC (2007) Occupational Health: Dealing With the Issues: A TUC Education Workbook for Union Reps, TUC, London, available at www.unionlearn.org.uk/extrasUL/education/occupationalhealth.pdf (accessed 3 February 2009)

Worldwatch Institute (2008) State of the World 2008: Innovations for a Sustainable Economy, Worldwatch Institute, Washington DC

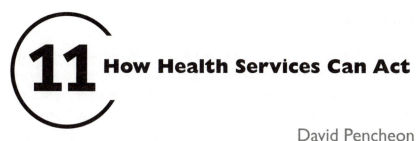

11 How Health Services Can Act

David Pencheon

The credit crunch is about borrowing from our children; the climate crunch is about stealing from them.

David Pencheon

Summary

Every health service in every country has the responsibility and opportunity to set an important example about how the needs of today's populations can be met, without compromising the ability to meet the needs of populations tomorrow. Climate change is the biggest risk faced by health organizations – and all other organizations. The appropriate language is therefore of 'resilience', 'risk management' and 'organizational survival'. In the short term improving energy efficiency can save both money and carbon. But efficiency improvements will not be enough; it will be transformational change of care pathways that will reduce activity to ensure big carbon reductions. Costs must be measured in terms of carbon as well as money. Active travel and improving the food served by health services can save money, reduce carbon emissions and improve health – the triple bottom line. Procurement of goods and commissioning of services are very important ways of reducing the indirect carbon footprint of health care organizations. Carbon footprints need to be measured, corporately owned and reported. Carbon governance needs to become as important as financial and clinical governance. Health organizations have huge scope for reputational gain from wide-ranging action on climate change.

You may wish to read this chapter in conjunction with Chapter 10, about how health practitioners can work with other types of organizations, which has more information on travel planning (including walking and cycling), food, sustainable events and workplace health and climate change.

Key terms

Carbon literacy: General knowledge or awareness of the concepts, causes and effects of greenhouse gases.

Carbon numeracy: Knowledge and skills to participate in carbon trading systems, financial incentives etc.

Direct carbon emissions: Energy use from buildings from combustion of fossil fuels, e.g. gas for heating and hot water.

Indirect carbon emissions: The carbon associated with procurement and transport, use and disposal of products and services.

Double bottom line: Simultaneous financial and social return on investment (e.g. saving money and health improvement).

Triple bottom line: Simultaneous financial, social and environmental return on investment (e.g. saving money, health improvement and mitigating climate change).

Risk management: The process of assessing risks and taking steps either to eliminate or reduce them; usually involves the regular updating of a risk register.

Introduction

The role of health services appears simple: to provide accessible, cost-effective, safe and appropriate care to meet the planned and unplanned needs of a population. What often gets forgotten is the role of health services to prevent illness and promote health. Every health service in every country has the responsibility and opportunity to set an important example about how organizations and individuals could and should behave to meet the needs of today's population without compromising the ability to meet the needs of populations tomorrow.

Health care is a very here and now activity. We are all focused on giving and receiving the best possible care this very day, this very hour and sometimes this very minute. To do this to the best of our abilities *and* to be concerned about future years and decades is a huge challenge. In trying to address the enormity of climate change, it is important for health practitioners to remember that, initially, we will be most effective through our own efforts and the efforts of others. This will require a lot of persuasion and demonstration that doing today's job as well as possible is not incompatible – indeed is usually highly congruent – with the delivery of high quality health care tomorrow.

To do this, there are crucial skills, techniques and knowledge that a health practitioner must have or develop – which are referred to throughout this book – in addition to huge commitment. As in all campaigns demonstrating the need for profound and urgent change, this will involve sacrifices, accusations and tough decisions. However, the goal – decarbonizing the world, and ensuring a future for the next generations – could not be more worthwhile.

This chapter is about how individual practitioners can shape the health organizations of which they are a part. Changing health services will not happen overnight and is taking place in the face of vested interests and opposition. Failure to understand the barriers and constraints will surely lead health practitioners to become frustrated and lose momentum and focus. This is particularly difficult when we know that the time we have left to decarbonize significantly all human activities is probably much shorter than most people realize – including senior decision-makers in health care systems. Health practitioners finally got the message about tobacco control in many western countries, but it took far too long.

Words matter

Campaigns about climate change often refer to environmental impact, green alternatives and actions to help 'save the planet'. The words 'environment', 'green' and 'planet' are not necessarily the best to use to convince people who are working to tight operational deadlines. As in all good communication, empathy is the key.

Changing health care services, like changing any organization, is about convincing those in power and authority that the risk of making significant and often transformational change is less than the risk of not doing so. Unless your health care system is blessed with truly outstanding leadership, and these leaders have some unusually powerful executive authority, you will need – over time – to get over half of all senior people in the organization genuinely on board. They need to understand that climate change is the biggest risk the organization faces. At the time of writing, most organizational leaders, executive and non-executive, would not agree with this view. This is not because they are short-sighted or selfish.

It is because the evidence has not been communicated powerfully enough in terms that are alarming but not defeatist. (Is it serious? Yes! Can we do something about it? Yes!) And the words that need to be used are not 'environment', 'green' and 'planet'. They are 'resilience', 'risk management' and 'organizational survival'. The methods by which we meet the fundamental objectives of health care services need to be re-articulated in ways that make sense in a lower-carbon world.

There are three main reasons that health practitioners can bring to bear to create organizational change (Pencheon, 2009).

Firstly there are potentially big savings to be made (cost, tax, reputation...) and there is a need for energy resilience and robustness. This is likely to be the most important reason for senior management (see below).

Secondly, health services have a special responsibility and opportunity to lead by example. When health services and health practitioners take issues seriously, such as tobacco control and climate change, then this sends out an important message to the public.

Thirdly, there is very good evidence from the UK of willingness and commitment from health service workers and health professionals that addressing such important health threats as climate change is part of the core business of health services and systems. 'Promoting and protecting health is a core duty of health services, no matter how funded and organized. Adapting to, and mitigating, climate change are therefore a core part of the role of health services' (Pencheon, 2009).

However, there are three additional reasons for health practitioners to take action to change the health system of which they are a part (Pencheon, 2009):

- In many countries there will be legally mandated targets.
- There is a strong scientific evidence base regarding the causes of climate change (often stronger than the evidence we use as clinicians to diagnose and treat).

- Lastly, there are many opportunities for immediate health benefits for individuals, health care systems and whole societies (see Chapter 4).

Potentially big savings in big organizations

There is nothing better to engage managers and clinicians in health services than to be able to demonstrate savings of resources (especially money) that can be redirected to patient care.

Saving money will give you confidence that a difference can be made and crucially it will give the senior executive teams of health organizations confidence to act. It is easier to take the more radical, transformational and strategic steps that are needed in system reform to reduce carbon emissions by 80 per cent when people are comfortable with the initial less ambitious steps. Even if they are sceptical about climate change, it will be difficult to ignore the potential savings that can be made from taking action on energy efficiency or reducing demand or minimizing waste.

However, although increasing efficiency is an attractive way to engage many clinicians and managers, it is only an early milestone on the way to more profound changes in behaviour and culture. Reducing activity (such as delivering fewer episodes of care) is much more effective in addressing climate change and will result in much greater savings. It is difficult to sell reduced activity in health services. Most health systems around the world contain strong inbuilt incentives to increase activity. This can be either due to systems that depend on fee for service, or on systems that are performance measured and managed through activity (relatively easy) rather than outcome (relatively difficult).

Box 11.1
Kentish Town Integrated Care Centre (Camden Primary Care Trust)

This new centre has been developed with sustainability in mind from beginning to end:

- onsite reclamation of demolished building materials;
- retention of trees and incorporation of a garden seen from the waiting area into the design (positive effect on mental well-being);
- natural lighting and ventilation strategy, using solar power;
- high levels of thermal insulation;
- no patient parking except for disabled people;
- four charging points for pooled use electric vehicles in the staff car park;
- 38 cycle racks with weather protection; staff showers to encourage cycling to work;
- high efficiency in terms of space allocation; hot desking; multiple use rooms (including GP consultation rooms);
- extensive health promotion activity within the community incorporated to address health inequalities and reduce the numbers of primary care presentations at acute trusts.

Source: Community Health Partnerships (2008)

Total carbon impact matters

What is needed is transformational reform of systems and pathways that really address climate change. Not: 'how do make this make this planned new hospital really efficient?' But: 'can we really afford the carbon impact of this brand new hospital; are there really no lower-carbon patient pathways that deliver an equivalent quality of patient care?'

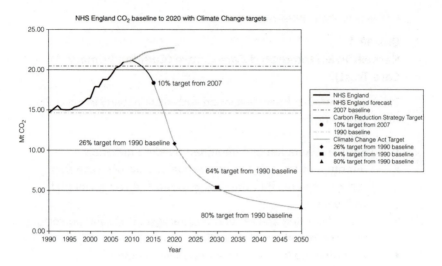

Figure 11.1 NHS England CO$_2$ baseline to 2020 with climate change targets

Source: NHS Sustainable Development Unit (2009)

In England, the National Health Service (NHS) has a carbon footprint of 18 million tonnes of CO$_2$ per year. This is composed of energy (22 per cent), travel (18 per cent) and procurement (60 per cent). Despite greater carbon efficiency, the NHS has increased its carbon footprint by 40 per cent since 1990 – see Figure 11.1. This means that meeting the Climate Change Act target of a 34 per cent reduction by 2020 will be a huge challenge (NHS Sustainable Development Unit, 2009).

The key issue is the absolute impact of health services. There is no point in having more efficient hospitals and health care systems if there are more of them or they are bigger, or both. New buildings (if they are in addition to old buildings, rather than replacing them) will always increase the carbon footprint of a health care system regardless of how efficient they are – hence the need to decommission redundant buildings and services. Reducing overall levels of activity (episodes of care) is the most effective way to mitigate climate change.

The challenge for health practitioners is to get as many of their colleagues and senior leaders in the system aware of three variables:

- quality of health care;
- cost of delivering health care in terms of money;
- cost of delivering health care in terms of carbon.

It is valuable to model savings in terms of a well-understood metric that finance officers, planners and chief executives can understand immediately, such as 'return on investment'. This is dependent on current and future rates of interest and, of course, discounting rates used in valuing future benefits. If a scheme to save both energy and money (e.g. ultra efficient lighting or hospital-wide heat insulation) is proposed where the return on investment is, for instance, two years, one way to sell this investment is to make it clear that after two years without such an investment, money will be lost that could be going straight to patient care, and the opportunity to mitigate climate change has also been lost.

Initiatives to increase efficiency and save money therefore contribute to a double bottom line: both saving money and mitigating climate change. However, because of the possibility of immediate health benefits (see below and Chapter 4) there is often the possibility of a *triple* bottom line: saving money, mitigating climate change and improving immediate health. The improved health may relate to those participating (for example, more active travel by staff, patients and visitors, through the direct benefits of increasing levels of regular physical activity, should improve physical and mental health), but also to the population at large if the same interventions reduce the levels of air pollution or road-related trauma.

Examples of immediate savings: Double bottom line

The best examples of immediate savings come from increased energy efficiency of heating, cooling, ventilation and hot water. Generation on site using a combined heat and power (CHP) plant is an obvious example. And if this can help with the laundry, sterilization and incineration, the benefits will be even greater.

Box 11.2
Combined heat and power (CHP) scheme at Birmingham Heartlands & Solihull NHS Trust

The CHP scheme enables the hospital to generate its own electricity in a purpose-designed energy centre. The electricity is generated from a gas-powered engine and the heat comes from hot water. Combining the two creates the carbon saving. Rather than relying on separate boilers to heat water for the central heating systems, the buildings connected to the energy network exploit the heat the engine generates as it produces electricity.

This project was part of a £5 million energy efficiency programme that is recording savings of £688,000 a year and cutting emissions of carbon by 1627 tonnes per year – the equivalent of a forest of 2503 trees – as well as reducing other harmful green house gases such as sulphur dioxide.

Source: NHS Sustainable Development Unit (2009)

CHP and other related technologies such as District Heating and Hot Water systems are not new. There are other emerging technologies that health practitioners have the perfect opportunity to share across a whole building and even a whole system. Examples include ultra efficiency lighting using, light emitting diodes (LEDs). Newer forms of lighting ensure that nearly all the electrical energy gets converted into light and not into heat. (A crude test of such technology is that the colder the light is to touch carefully, the more efficient it is likely to be.)

Making progress is usually not dependent on the rapid advance of technology but on another equally important science: how to change people and organizations. A valuable technique is gain-sharing: sharing the money saved by – for example – everyone switching off unnecessary lights, between all staff who control the lights.

Triple bottom line: Adding in health benefits

Besides the double bottom line of saving money *and* acting on climate change, there is a third bottom line of immediate improved psychological and physical health. Nearly all the behaviour changes that we encourage to mitigate climate change in the health care system will have both immediate and future benefits for third parties; examples include travel and food.

Travel, transport and access

Approximately 20 per cent of a health organization's carbon footprint is likely to be related to the transport of staff, patients and visitors. The NHS accounts for 5 per cent of all road traffic in England (NHS Confederation, 2007). There is a strong 'triple bottom line' business case for a sustainable travel plan (Department for Transport, 2008; Griffiths and Stewart, 2009).

Financial savings

- savings in reimbursed car mileage;
- productivity improvements from staff time saved in travel (tele conferencing, videoconferencing, homeworking);
- avoiding land purchase or costs of building and maintaining car parks.

Operational benefits

- improved access for patients, visitors and deliveries;
- reducing staff time on problems causes by parking shortages.

Human resources

- improved staff retention, a more attractive recruitment package, reduction in staff sick days through better staff health, improved staff morale, better home-life balance.

Corporate social responsibility

- reduced carbon emissions;
- benefits to community relations from contribution to reducing congestion, pollution and road traffic accidents;
- can assist when making planning applications to expand premises.

As discussed in Chapter 4, the health benefit – creating the triple bottom line business case – is that increased levels of physical activity will have multiple health benefits for both those directly participating (reduced risk of coronary heart disease, obesity, diabetes, minor mental illness, etc.) but also for others through reduced air pollution and less road-related trauma.

A travel plan means so much more than just one cycle rack behind the rubbish bins – rather it means a set of cycle racks highly visible and closer to the front door than the non-disabled car parking spaces. There should be good quality washing facilities, storage and clothes drying facilities too. All health care facilities in which you work need to have easy access to car sharing/pooling opportunities. Not everyone will be able to use public transport, so people should be rewarded who use car share schemes, the organization of which is made much easier by the use of the internet (see for example www.liftshare. com). Car pooling can be incentivized by rewarding multi-occupancy car use with reserved spaces and reduced charges.

We must overturn inverse reimbursement schemes that financially reward high-emission cars. Financial incentives should work directly against higher-carbon transport options, with rewards for active travel (e.g. cycling and walking) and

Box 11.3
Winchester and Eastleigh Healthcare NHS Trust Travel Plan

The NHS Trust has introduced a patient travel bus saving 4000 patient journeys per annum, equating to a reduction of 68,000 miles. This has been combined with a staff travel plan that has reduced staff car journeys by 1540 per week. Based on an estimation of 8 miles per journey this equates to 500,000 miles per annum saved.

The Trust will shortly offer staff who cycle to work a free 'Loan-U-Lock' security system to help protect them from bike theft. Both of these initiatives have led to a reduction in the number of cars travelling to the Royal Hampshire County Hospital site.

Source: NHS Sustainable Development Unit (2009)

lower-carbon methods of mechanized transport (e.g. public transport, car sharing and low-emission cars). For both staff and visitors, good directions can be put on your website that give all the lower carbon options first and their exact use, cost, timing, limitations and maps (Sustrans (2006) provides good advice).

We should support nurses and doctors and other staff with decent low-cost accommodation at or near their place of work, so that they do not have to spend both carbon and long hours on travel.

Food served by health services

Health organizations are often the biggest buyers of food and preparers of meals across a population. They have the opportunity to serve fresh and seasonal food, investing in local economies, reducing the carbon footprint

Box 11.4
Cornwall NHS Food Programme, Central Food Production Unit

The Central Food Production Unit provides high-quality meals, sourced mainly from local produce, to the Royal Cornwall, St Michaels' and West Cornwall Hospitals. The Unit is the culmination of many years of work by a public-private-government partnership and is an excellent example of innovative public procurement. It meets the following 'triple bottom line' objectives:

- reduction in food miles (and therefore carbon emissions);
- provision of healthy, balanced meals for patients, staff and visitors and a wide range of special needs diets;
- sourcing and cooking on a tight budget;
- guaranteeing local farmers, fishermen and food producers year-round orders for their high-quality products;
- potential for business expansion outside of the health care environment, e.g. catering for other organizations;
- partnerships with local colleges for catering students.

Source: Community Health Partnerships (2008)

associated with food purchasing, preparation and serving. Reducing meat in the diet is another example of a health benefit (see Chapter 4 for a description of the impact of high consumption of meat on both health and greenhouse gas emissions).

The power of large organizations to influence staff, patients and visitors

Health services are big, and therefore have the ability to influence a huge number of staff (the NHS employs over 1.3 million people) and also those who use the health service – and the families and friends of both these groups. However, being big (especially with little competition and/or state protection) risks the potential incentives to taking genuine action being dwarfed by the day-to-day pressures of running a risk-averse health care system.

Health practitioners need to be able to find ways of influencing an organization whose scope and complexity can constrain their freedom to act. As argued in Chapter 5, health professionals, especially those that have front-line contact with the public, command an important and valuable respect both within the health service and beyond.

There are many points at which practitioners can influence the organization. An executive or a non-executive on the board clearly has huge responsibility to ensure all decisions are taken with the fully informed knowledge of the likely consequences of and for climate change.

Each and every member of staff can practice personally what needs to be done by all of us (see Chapter 7), in the obvious areas such as energy use, transport, contracting and buying, and the redesign of buildings, and clinical pathways.

Design of buildings

Buildings are one of the most important causes of the carbon-intensity of care pathways. Constructing new buildings therefore presents unique opportunities for shaping the way health care is delivered. Everything possible must be done to ensure the building is constructed and operable in a low-carbon way and stimulates climate-friendly behaviour by all its users: highly energy efficient, passively cooled, efficiently lit, stairs more visible than elevators.

Box 11.5
The Plowright Medical Centre, Swaffham, Norfolk

The Plowright Surgery in Norfolk was built for a general practitioner patient population of 5200 patients. It sets a new energy benchmark for surgeries and uses just 54kWh of electricity and 90kWh of gas per m² per year. This energy use is far below the Department of Health's standard for new buildings.

The design of the building ensures effective use of natural light and ventilation, without air-conditioning. The carbon dioxide emissions of the building are only 31 tonnes per year (the equivalent of about three people's carbon emissions per year in the United Kingdom).

The cost of the building fell within the lowest quartile of the funding criteria (at £1706 per m²), proving that low carbon does not have to cost more.

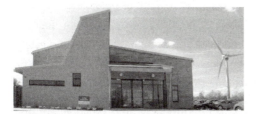

Figure 11.2 The Plowright Medical Centre, Swaffam, Norfolk

Source: NHS Sustainable Development Unit (2009)

Once a building has been designed there is much less opportunity to incorporate a radically lower carbon footprint into it retrospectively. Many of the buildings we use in health care systems today will still be with us in 20–30 years.

Procurement of goods and commissioning of services

Only limited research has been carried out on the carbon intensity of health services and systems around the world. What research has been done (Sustainable Development Commission et al, 2008) suggests that over half of the carbon footprint of a health system can be attributed to the buying and disposal of products. Health practitioners who have any influence on procurement need to ensure that all contracts make it clear that suppliers are expected to have a genuine commitment to acting on climate change. Contracts need to be negotiated so that this influence is perpetuated right down the supply chain. Initially, this will only be possible in words, but as soon as possible contracting and commissioning needs to be climate sensitive in ways that are quantifiable. Only when contracts are not renewed and a competitive culture is established (often through clear and open reporting) will the whole supply chain be focused on actions necessary to mitigate climate change.

Here are four examples of phrases to be introduced into procurement and commissioning contracts:

- 'This service/hospital/health care organization does not do business with organizations that cannot demonstrate a genuine, practical and measurable approach to sustainability and climate change.'
- 'Criteria relating to sustainability and low-carbon operations will increasingly be used in the commissioning of services and the procuring of goods.'
- 'Each year/cycle we will increase the weighting given to your qualitative and quantitative commitment to a sustainable and lower-carbon health service.'
- 'Systematic plans to monitor and reduce your carbon impact and improve sustainability will be a highly significant criterion on which your tender will be judged.'

You can't manage what you can't measure!

Carbon is usually chosen as the key metric of understanding, quantifying and addressing climate change. The other dimensions of sustainable development, corporate social responsibly and good corporate citizenship referred to elsewhere in this chapter and in this book are more complex than the carbon impact of a person, a ward, a patient pathway, a hospital or a complete health care system.

Carbon measurement is crucially important in creating system and organizational change. Many senior leaders (and especially senior and middle managers in health services) are driven, managed and held accountable by what is measurable. Carbon dioxide equivalent (see Chapter 1 for explanation) is the term frequently used to summarize the greenhouse gases that are ultimately compromising everyone's health.

As health organizations get serious about climate change and sustainable development, the key issue is not just to act, but to demonstrate and monitor action through measurement. Although what gets measured also gets managed, it is equally likely that what gets measured gets manipulated. Explicitness and honesty in method, and a balance between both process and outcome measures, and a balance between numeric and narrative detail (with a core set of agreed and valid measurements that allow comparison) is needed.

Comparison is particularly important as it stimulates healthy and productive competition in the workplace – galvanizing individual and team action. It also gives the regulatory and legislative process some evidence on the most meaningful indicators and metrics for use across the system (NHS Institute for Innovation and Development, 2008).

Carbon footprinting is an increasingly important technique. The most important distinction currently is between a direct carbon footprint (defined as the carbon emissions from direct energy use: coal, gas, oil, etc. for heating, hot water, ventilation, cooling) and a total (direct and indirect) carbon footprint. The indirect carbon footprint is that generated through, for instance, travel and procurement. All definitions differ slightly, so clarity and openness about methodology are crucial when comparing between and within organizations.

Carbon literacy and numeracy

Being corporately socially responsible about the effect of organizational behaviour on climate means having a much greater understanding of carbon emissions, where they come from, how they can be reduced, how they are measured and their effects on the cost-effective delivery of safe health care.

Carbon literacy means being able to describe carbon cycles and some of the technologies that are being increasingly employed to address climate change at an organizational level. Carbon numeracy means being able to measure, monitor and compare consequences and actions. More details of carbon literacy and numeracy can be found in Chapters 1 and 7.

Performance monitoring and management

Inevitably, the subject of standards and criteria will arise when considering performance management. As time is short to take the necessary action to reduce runaway climate change, the best possible should be the benchmark. The predominant policy should be: 'we cannot afford to build care pathways and buildings that are not as climate friendly and low carbon as they can possibly be'. Any other option should be considered as risky and ultimately dangerous.

The UK Government's policy is to achieve an 80 per cent reduction in carbon emissions by 2050. The NHS is setting itself an initial target of a 10 per cent reduction on 2007 levels by 2015, which is a real challenge given the current upward trajectory of emissions – see Figure 11.1 (NHS Sustainable Development Unit, 2009).

Corporate ownership and governance

Taking action on climate change in health care systems, as within any system, has so far largely been the preserve of pressure groups and personal advocacy. Due to increasing social awareness, scientific evidence, staff pressure and international governmental regulation and taxation, health care systems around the world are starting to understand the need to address climate change as a corporate issue. The 'greatest health challenge' has to be a central issue in organizational objectives and risk management within health care organizations.

The most compelling reason to act (after the business case for many immediate tasks, such as energy efficiency) is that climate change is a huge and very real risk to human health, and human health is the core business of health services. This means acknowledging the risks, opportunities, barriers and consequences explicitly in everything corporate, from the constitution of the organization to its risk management process. The aim is to ensure that climate change is not perceived and thus treated as a side issue to consider when everything else is sorted, but as a central part of the day job.

Most organizational and employment policies and procedures were written, consulted upon and agreed well before climate change was shown to be a serious issue. Most, if not all, policies will need to be revisited. Staff representatives and unions can lobby for climate-friendly policies for the workplace as part of workplace health, for example regarding transport (see Chapter 10 for more information).

Embedding reduction of greenhouse gas emissions as a top priority in an organization needs the usual array of managerial and organizational commitments, such as:

- Include climate change as a cross-cutting issue (in the same way as equality and diversity issues are often handled) in all policies and strategies.
- All policies, strategies, programme and project plans should include an evaluation of their impact on carbon emissions and be carbon-proofed, that is, no proposal should result in an increase in carbon emissions and all should make some contribution towards the agreed target reduction.
- All staff, from the chief executive outwards, should have a personal objective relating to sustainability in their job descriptions, specifications or job plans. It should be asked about at interviews and appraisals.
- Learning opportunities should be provided to enable staff to develop their knowledge and competence on sustainability and climate change strategies. It should be regularly discussed in staff meetings.
- Climate change ultimately threatens all organizations' survival and should therefore be included on the risk register, with regular monitoring of action plans to reduce greenhouse gas emissions by risk management and audit committees.

- All health organizations should make strong links with the emergency planning system for both adaptation and mitigation of climate change (see Chapter 12).

Box 11.6
Climate change risk management

- Physical risks: direct impacts of climate change, e.g. extreme weather events.
- Regulatory risks: tightening national and international regulations.
- Competitive risks: not meet customer expectations.
- Reputation risks: perceived lack of action.
- Operational risks: from rising energy prices, energy insecurity etc.

Source: www.climategroup.org

Public visibility and reputational gain

The huge opportunity open to health care systems is their public visibility. Just as many people only took tobacco harm seriously when doctors stopped smoking (see Chapter 5), the public may well only take climate change seriously when health care organizations take it seriously (and are *seen* to do so). The public reporting of action on climate change is therefore very important. Many initiatives are introduced into hospitals that are highly effective but largely invisible. More innovations that are visible to patients and the public are needed. Ultra efficient lighting using light emitting diodes that are motion sensitive is one example; generation of power through using medium size to large wind turbines where feasible is another. Health services can influence the public, as well as the public influencing them.

For instance, on health service publications you can state: 'This publication is printed on fully recycled paper, forestry stewardship certified, post-consumer waste and chlorine free. Inks are vegetable-based and coatings are water-based.' All health care premises should have a highly visible notice (e.g. in their

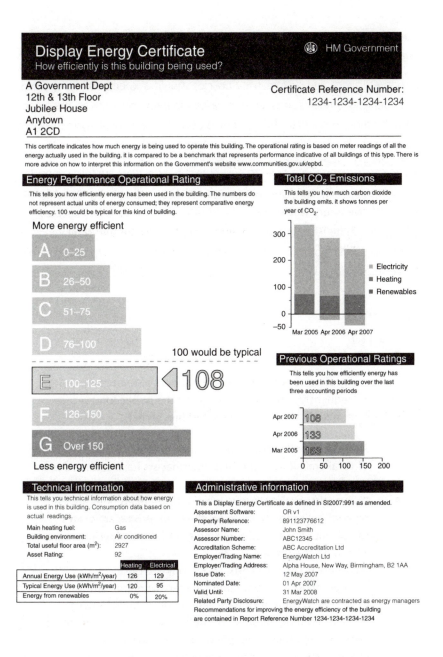

Figure 11.3 Mock-up of Display Energy Certificate for building energy performance

reception or waiting area) of their carbon efficiency against a nationally or internationally recognized scale – see Figure 11.3 for example.

Carbon efficiency and sustainability policies should also be publicly reported, for example in annual reports. Press releases and media briefings on the organization's actions on climate change should be undertaken regularly, in the same way as other aspects of patient and population safety.

Health care organizations need to ensure that their actions are fully supported by the local population. Addressing climate change will become an ever-more important civic issue, where hospital and other premises will be expected not only to contribute to adaption and mitigation, but also be seen to leading the agenda wherever possible. The reputational benefit to a health care commissioner or provider taking action on climate change is considerable.

Box 11.7
Towards low-carbon community pharmacy

Community pharmacies form an integral part of their community and are frequently visited by members of the public (on average in England people visit a pharmacy 14 times a year).

- Pharmaceutical products are responsible for 22 per cent of total emissions in the NHS. Pharmacists have systems for the disposal of unused medicines.
- Pharmacists in the UK give prescription-linked brief advice on healthy living; in doing so, they can also be advocates for greener lifestyles, for example walking and cycling more and using the car less.
- Pharmacists can save costs, show they are business entrepreneurs and community leaders who are contributing to efforts to combat climate change by installing energy-efficient lighting, improving insulation, heating and cooling systems – and telling people what they have done.
- Pharmacists can sign-post people to local 'green' events and provide information for people on reducing their carbon emissions.

Source: Pharmacy HealthLink (2008)

The time is coming when health care organizations will compete to advertize their achievements in corporate social responsibility. In systems where the public really can exercise informed choice, the corporate social responsibility credentials of a health care organization will soon be a deciding factor.

An especially powerful method of stimulating innovative practice in the early days of a movement before it becomes absolutely mainstream and corporate is through highly public praising using awards. National and regional award schemes are developing, but health organizations can develop their own internal award systems to recognize the achievements of both individual champions and teams. This can be a very cost-effective and highly visible way of sharing properly evaluated effective practice and rewarding individuals and organizations that have excelled. It would be useful to share failures as well because the learning can be enormous, but we are sadly not always willing to share their failures in public.

Climate change as part of a wider set of global challenges

Finally, as a health practitioner, do not become too single-minded about advocating climate change. It is one of the most serious health challenges facing us globally, probably the most serious. But it is not the only health challenge. It can valuably be embedded within the wider set of serious global health issues, ranging from climate change to obesity, to international inequities in wealth and opportunity, to wars over natural resources.

The decision is not which is the most important. These issues are all intimately related and the solution to any one of them is supportive and interrelated with the solutions for the rest. To date, international poverty, inequity and discrimination have caused far more deaths than climate change. Poorer countries have much lower carbon emissions. The silver lining to the global challenge of climate change is that many of the potential solutions to this issue may also help to solve others. For further discussion of these issues, see Chapter 5.

Conclusion

Climate change is happening on our watch and will be our legacy. Health care systems and the practitioners who work within them have special responsibilities and opportunities. If we do not take this opportunity to act right now, our children and grandchildren will have every right to look in amazement at our selfishness and lack of courage. Follies of history are often borne out of ignorance. There is no ignorance here – that means an even greater folly if we do not make rapid progress.

Action points

1   Are you aware of a number of potential technologies to reduce your team's or department's carbon footprint? Can you routinely ask why a particular carbon-reducing technology is not being considered across the whole building or the whole discipline or the whole system?

2   How can you measure quality of health care more on outcomes (current and future) and less on activity rates, both to improve health and to substantially reduce carbon emissions?

3   Can you articulate your plans for action on climate change in terms of money saved, using a process such as 'return on investment'?

4   Can you go a step further and articulate immediate action in terms of a triple bottom line: health improvement, mitigation of climate change and saving money?

5   Is there any potential for gain-sharing (sharing savings) in your team, directorate or department?

6   Is the reporting of the progress of the health care system of which you are a part made public regularly and clearly, so that you gain the best possible reputation for your leadership on tackling climate change?

7   Are you involved in designing care pathways or new buildings? If so, ensure that the climate and carbon consequences are incorporated from the very beginning.

8   Are you involved in buying and contracting? If so, ensure that statements about carbon reduction and sustainable development are specified in all contracts.

9   Are you in a position to lobby for the development of a comprehensive travel plan at board level? In particular can you lobby for travel remuneration systems that incentivize low-carbon modes of transport?

10 Can you influence all the policies and plans with which you are involved to ensure that their impact on carbon emissions is evaluated and that they are carbon-proofed (that is, that they do not add to the carbon emissions of your organization)?

11 Can you suggest that action on climate change and sustainable development is included as a cross-cutting issue in job descriptions, job interviews, personal objectives and appraisals, risk registers, induction events, staff meetings etc.?

References

Camden Primary Care Trust (2008) 'Kentish Town: How the New LIFT Development for Camden Primary Care Trust meets the Sustainability Agenda', available at www.communityhealthpartnerships.co.uk/?ob=1&id=75 (accessed 2 February 2009)

Community Health Partnerships (2008) 'Innovative Production Unit Supplying Local Food to Hospitals, 1st July 2008', available at www.communityhealthpartnerships.co.uk/index.php?id=87&ob=2 (accessed 2 February 2009)

Department for Transport (2008) 'The Essential Guide to Travel Planning', available at www.dft.gov.uk/pgr/sustainable/travelplans/work/essentialguide.pdf (accessed 2 February 2009)

Griffiths, J. and Stewart, L. (2009) *Sustaining a Healthy Future: taking action on climate change*, 2nd edition, Faculty of Public Health and NHS Sustainable Development Unit and NHS Confederation

NHS Confederation (2007) 'Taking the temperature – Towards an NHS response to global warming', NHS Confederation, London

NHS Institute for Innovation and Development (2008) 'The Good Indicators Guide: Understanding how to Choose and Use Indicators', available at www.apho.org.uk/resource/item.aspx?RID=44584 (accessed 2 February 2009)

NHS Sustainable Development Unit (2009) 'Saving carbon, improving health: NHS carbon reduction strategy for England', Office of the Strategic Health Authorities, England, available at www.sdu.nhs.uk

Pencheon, D. (2009) 'Health services and climate change: what can be done?', editorial, *Journal of Health Services Research and Policy*, vol 14, no 1, pp2–4

Pharmacy HealthLink (2008) 'Our Planet', available at www.pharmacymeetspubli-chealth.org.uk/pdf/Our-Planet.pdf (accessed 3 February 2009)

Sustainable Development Commission, Stockholm Environment Institute, NHS Sustainable Development Unit (2008) 'NHS England Carbon Emissions: carbon footprint study', NHS Sustainable Development Unit, London, available at www. sdu.nhs.uk (accessed 21 July 2009)

Sustrans (2006) 'How to produce active travel directions', available at www. sustrans.org.uk/webfiles/AT/Publications/June%202006%20-How%20to%20 produce%20active%20travel%20travel%20directions%20.pdf (accessed 2 February 2009)

12 How to Prepare for the Health Effects of Climate Change

Giovanni Leonardi

Adaptation is the only response available for the impacts that will occur over the next several decades before mitigation measures can have an effect.

Nicholas Stern (2007)
The Economics of Climate Change

Summary

Adaptation to climate change is likely to reduce expected impacts on health in two ways: firstly, by requiring changes in the roles of health agencies, including planning and response to extreme weather events and surveillance of infectious disease; and secondly, by modifications in non-health sectors, that is, food production, transport, built environment. Who is competent to take these actions? Nobody can state with confidence that they are. However, much of the competence and skills that have been applied to previous health challenges can be applied to facilitating a transition to a society adapted to climate change.

Each and every practitioner can make an essential contribution to adaptation to climate change. As educated professionals, we have the capacity to integrate much information relevant to prevention of health impacts of climate change. As practitioners in contact with members of the public, we can influence and support their behaviour concerning actions that might protect them and their families from the consequences of climate change. Health practitioners can also support each other in both these roles. Overall, the health community can promote the increased resilience of their local community to adapt to climate change. This chapter aims to give you guidance on how.

Key terms

Capacity: A combination of all the strengths and resources available within a community, society or organization that can reduce the level of risk, or the effects of a disaster.

Complementarity: The interrelationship of adaptation and mitigation whereby the outcome of one supplements or depends on the outcome of the other.

Critical facilities: The primary physical structures, technical facilities and systems that are socially, economically or operationally essential to the functioning of a society or community, both in routine circumstances and in the extreme circumstances of an emergency.

Disaster: A serious disruption of the functioning of a community or a society involving widespread human, material, economic or environmental losses and impacts, which exceeds the ability of the affected community or society to cope using its own resources.

Early warning system: The set of capacities needed to generate and disseminate timely and meaningful warning information to enable individuals, communities and organizations threatened by a hazard to prepare and to act appropriately and in sufficient time to reduce the possibility of harm or loss.

Emergency management: The organization and management of resources and responsibilities for dealing with all aspects of emergencies, in particular preparedness, response and rehabilitation.

Extreme weather event: An event that is rare at a particular place (obviously, the characteristics of what is called 'extreme weather' may vary from place to place, but typically may include floods and droughts).

Mainstreaming: The integration of policies and measures to address climate change in ongoing sector-based and development planning and decision-making.

Relief/response: The provision of assistance or intervention during or immediately after a disaster to meet the life preservation and basic subsistence needs of those people affected; it can be of immediate, short-term or protracted duration.

Resilience: The capacity of a system, community or society potentially exposed to hazards to adapt, by resisting or changing in order to reach and maintain an acceptable level of functioning and structure; this is determined by the degree to which the social system is capable of organizing itself to increase its capacity for learning from past disasters for better future protection.

Vulnerability: The characteristics and circumstances of a community, system or asset that make it susceptible to the damaging effects of a hazard.

Introduction

Responses to climate change have been classified according to whether they aim to reduce emissions of greenhouse gases (mitigation), or to reduce the impacts of ongoing and expected climate change on human communities (adaptation). Effective mitigation benefits not only human systems but also all natural systems (Semenza et al, 2008).

Figure 12.1 schematically illustrates the combined benefits of mitigation and adaptation activities, in terms of overall reduction of expected impacts.

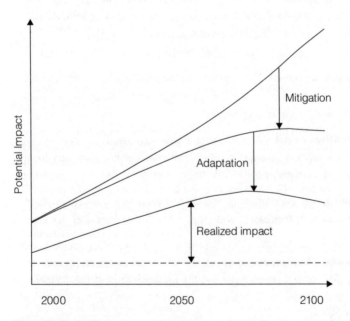

Figure 12.1 Adaptation and mitigation contribution to impact reduction (schematic)

Source: Author

In fact, the distinction is not always easy to apply in practice. Mitigation and adaptation do not happen independently. When one is implemented, the other can be affected in both favourable and adverse ways (Klein et al, 2007). Decisions on adaptation and mitigation are taken at different governance levels and interrelationships exist within and across each level. It is not yet possible to answer the question as to whether or not investment in adaptation would buy time for mitigation.

In public health terms, as we have seen in Chapters 4 and 5, mitigation of climate change is a prerequisite of avoiding the widening of health inequities globally. However, adaptive responses to climate change, while necessary, are a less sure way to reduce health inequities, since self-interested adaptation by those populations with most resources would increase the health gap (Friel et al, 2008).

Some actions can help foster both adaptation and mitigation, such as sustainable agricultural systems, soil and water conservation measures involving planting trees that then absorb greenhouse gases, or renewable energy initiatives.

Some have suggested that when interventions affect the hardware of human organization (energy systems, buildings, transport systems), they will be most effective when they are designed to achieve both mitigation and adaptation (Homer-Dixon, 2007). In this context, the term 'mainstreaming' describes the integration of policies and measures that integrate climate change into development planning and ongoing sector-based decision-making. The benefit of mainstreaming would be to ensure the sustainability of investments and to reduce the sensitivity of development activities to current and future climatic conditions (Klein et al, 2005). Although this approach seems reasonable, this chapter will include an overview of strategies for adaptation to climate change, including those that have not been designed with mitigation as an additional aim. Anyway, while adaptation action has become an unavoidable and indispensable complement to mitigation action, it is certainly not an alternative to the reducing greenhouse gases (GHG) emissions (EU Commission, 2007).

Are all these questions too much to comprehend at the same time and our capacity for reasonable action too small? Perhaps not! The main theme of this chapter is the idea of 'resilience'. Resilience has been defined as the state's capacity to absorb sudden shocks, to adapt to longer-term changes in socio-economic conditions and to sustainably resolve societal disputes without catastrophic breakdown. The opposite is 'brittleness' (Homer-Dixon, 2007). It has been argued powerfully that our rush towards greater efficiency has made our civilization brittle and vulnerable. The model strategy for increasing resilience is to increase redundancy and reduce unnecessary complexity – to maintain 'slack' in the system (Homer-Dixon, 2007). To manage climate change risk means being prepared for scenarios we know are unlikely to happen, but would be disastrous if they did. We do this all the time when we take out insurance: we are prepared for our house burning down and for our house not burning down.

Areas for action on adaptation

Climate change, an environmental health hazard of unprecedented scale and complexity, requires health practitioners to develop new ways of thinking, communicating and acting (Frumkin and McMichael, 2008). It necessitates thinking in terms of a sustained time frame and it needs a system approach beyond the current boundaries of the health sciences and health sector. Communicating about the risks posed by climate change requires messages that motivate constructive engagement rather than indifference, fear or despair. Actions that address climate change should offer a range of health, environmental and social benefits (Frumkin and McMichael, 2008).

The framework of primary, secondary and tertiary prevention may be useful for bringing health and other sectors together:

- Primary prevention includes health promotion and requires action on the determinants of health to prevent disease occurring.
- Secondary prevention is essentially the early detection of disease, accompanied by appropriate intervention, such as health promotion or treatment.
- Tertiary prevention aims to reduce the impact of the disease and promote quality of life through active rehabilitation.

In this framework, actions to adapt to climate change may be considered as 'secondary or tertiary prevention', whereas actions to limit climate change could be described as 'primary prevention'.

The World Health Organization (WHO) has proposed an agenda for research on climate change and public health (WHO, 2009). The WHO has recommended five research areas, listed here with a comment on their relevance to public health services.

Recommendation 1: Interactions of climate change with other health determinants and trends

The implication of this for public health services is that they would strive to identify effective measures to strengthen public health systems to address several environmental health risks, integrating adaptation to climate change with factors such as economic development, energy management, urbanization, conservation of water, soil and other natural capital resources that support human life and welfare, social impacts and access to care.

Recommendation 2: Direct and indirect effects of climate change

This proposal is a reminder that immediate effects of disease vector distribution, heatwaves, drought events and flooding, for example, should be addressed by public health services with due consideration of long-term trends on factors underlying these hazards. These include management of water resources and their indirect consequences on drought and flood trends, as well as related human conflicts. Hostility between human population groups could be reduced by explicit collaborative management of access to natural resources. Health practitioners have enormous experience in liaising with numerous stakeholders when promoting change to services.

Recommendation 3: Comparing effectiveness of short-term interventions

Short-term interventions by health services or others can be monitored using public health methods. For results to be applicable without delay, both the proposed intervention and evaluation method would benefit from intense exchange of information and coordination between service providers and researchers, when designing and interpreting an evaluation programme. Possible comparisons are between countries, such as heatwave plans in different European countries. By highlighting the value of approaches in different contexts, international comparisons may provide information of relevance to countries where evaluation research is not feasible.

Recommendation 4: Assessing health impact of policies of non-health sectors

There are benefits to health from climate mitigation interventions in non-health sectors (see Chapter 4). Further evidence on joint benefits is required. Public health services at national and regional level will need to assess the health impact of policy decisions made by non-health sectors addressing climate change, a task not as difficult as it may sound provided the relevant non-health sector is willing to address it in collaboration with public health agencies.

Recommendation 5: Strengthening public health systems to address health effects of climate change

General public health skills are the foundation of effective interventions to address climate change, just the same as any other challenge to health. While researchers work to document the most effective means of implementing integrated strategies that reduce threats to climate change, public health service providers can include adaptation to climate change in their mandate.

Basic public health functions in relation to climate change

The main public health functions required include the following (Kovats and Hajat, 2008; McMichael et al, 2008):

- Document and communicate the actuality of health risks. National and (appropriate) sub-national formal health risk assessments could be carried out to identify the main health risks, their likely chronology and vulnerable sub-populations.
- Anticipate the 'pressure points' where health impacts are most likely to appear and ensure there is a good, continuing, health-outcome surveillance in place.
- Develop methods of causal attribution, such that the public and policy-makers can be advised as to the plausible likely contribution of climate change to the impacts of otherwise 'natural' events (e.g. Hurricane Katrina; Europe's 2003 heatwave, ongoing droughts in several continents). This also requires appropriate handling and communication of the complex issue of uncertainty.

- Develop rationally targeted prevention (adaptive) strategies. Accrue experience and knowledge about the options for reducing risk. Evaluate these for specified populations/communities in terms of averted disease/death/disability burden and in terms of their costs and benefits.
- Commit to systematic updating of scenario-based (future) health risk assessments. This will assist the public and policy-makers' understanding of the likely future risks to health in response to future social and economic change.

The topic of adaptation, or 'rationally targeted prevention', is addressed mostly by the fourth of these five public health functions. This chapter will focus on this function and will outline some of the suggestions that have been made concerning adaptation to climate change and its health consequences. In particular, it will outline several adaptive strategies including the overall role of health agencies, specific activities in relation to extreme events and longer-term plans, the role of municipalities and an overview of public health competencies for adaptation to climate change.

Role of health agencies in adaptation

There are four groups of adaptations that may be considered specifically by health systems (Ebi et al, 2006):

1   Modifications of existing prevention strategies: responses to climate change affect all systems of human organization, therefore they are likely to be more effective if integrated into the day-to-day management of all sectors that could affect human health.
2   Translation of policies and knowledge from other countries.
3   Restoration of surveillance, maintenance and prevention programmes that have been weakened or abandoned due to financial considerations.
4   Development of new policies to address new threats.

At a time when resources for supporting adaptation strategies may be scarce, and the time available for developing and implementing these strategies is also scarce, we must share with the utmost openness all experience and knowledge about the available options. For the same reasons, it would seem also extremely desirable that any intervention would be accompanied by arrangements for its own evaluation, so that lessons learnt can be rapidly heeded and convincingly disseminated.

Health response to climate change needs to be based on the essential public health services (Frumkin et al, 2008). Strengthening existing public health approaches involves:

- public education;
- preventive programmes;
- surveillance of disease;
- forecasting future health risks.

It needs to be complemented by activities that extend beyond the health sector (McMichael et al, 2008):

- early warning systems;
- neighbourhood support schemes;
- climate-proofed housing design;
- urban planning;
- water catchment;
- farming practices;
- disaster preparedness.

Health systems to support management of extreme events

Enhanced disaster response preparedness

According to the UN International Strategy for Disaster Reduction (ISDR), a disaster is a serious disruption of the functioning of a community or a society involving widespread human, material, economic or environmental losses and impacts, which exceeds the ability of the affected community or society to cope using its own resources (ISDR, 2009).

Disasters are increasing in number and severity. International institutional frameworks to reduce disasters are being strengthened under United Nations supervision (Basher, 2006). The UN ISDR has produced recommendations (ISDR, 2008) relevant at international and national levels:

- Make adaptation to climate change a fundamental pillar of any post-Kyoto agreement.
- Ensure that disaster risk reduction and climate risk management are core elements of adaptation to climate change.
- Establish mechanisms to provide sufficient funding for adaptation to climate change and risk reduction, especially to protect the most vulnerable.
- Take immediate action to implement adaptation to climate change and risk reduction in vulnerable countries in the next three years.

At the World Conference on Disaster Reduction in Japan in 2005, an agreement was reached by participating countries on a 'Framework for Action 2005–2015: Building the Resilience of Nations and Communities to Disasters'. The Hyogo Framework for Action identified five priorities for action that formed the basis of national platforms for disaster reduction (ISDR, 2005):

- Ensure that disaster risk reduction is a national and a local priority with a strong institutional basis for implementation.
- Identify, assess and monitor disaster risks and enhance early warning.
- Use knowledge, innovation and education to build a culture of safety and resilience at all levels.
- Reduce the underlying risk factors.
- Strengthen disaster preparedness for effective response at all levels.

At national and local level, guidance has been prepared by several agencies for specific natural hazards and related extreme events. Good overviews are available of such specific guidance in relation to health impacts (Menne and Ebe, 2005), highlighting the fragmentary nature of the evidence and systems available when considered across the several hazards expected. Work is in progress to improve this situation rapidly. Resilience in response to any specific hazard can be enhanced by linking specific lessons with existing civil protection systems.

Sudden impact disasters can be seen as a continuous time sequence of five different phases (Noji, 1997), each phase lasting from seconds to months or years, and each merging into the other:

- non-disaster or inter-disaster phase;
- pre-disaster or warning phase;
- impact phase;
- emergency phase (also called relief or isolation phase);
- reconstruction or rehabilitation phase.

Vulnerability reduction programmes can be identified for all the types of extreme weather events expected to increased in frequency and severity with climate change, and will reduce susceptibility and increase resilience (Keim, 2008).

Health security aspects of climate change were recognized by the World Health Organization (WHO, 2008a) and national security aspects of the environmental crises have also been identified. A convergence of objectives between health and civil protection activities could lead to fruitful developments in intervention design, implementation and evaluation.

The next section provides a brief overview of evidence for interventions in relation to adaptation to specific hazards.

Heatwaves

Climate change will increase the frequency and the intensity of heatwaves (see Chapter 2), and a range of measures, including improvements to housing, management of chronic diseases and institutional care of the elderly and the vulnerable, will need to be developed to reduce health impacts (Kovats and Hajat, 2008). Following the European heatwave of 2003, several projects have been conducted to estimate health impacts, factors affecting vulnerability of populations and physical infrastructure and a framework for preparedness and response. This effort has resulted in the production of guidance for the intro-duction and development of heat-health action plans (WHO, 2008b) and links to national plans. The principles identified are:

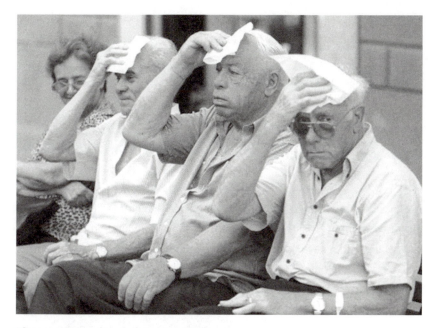

Figure 12.2 Italian heatwave, 2008

Source: Ansa, Italy (available at http://gallery.panorama.it/gallery/cronaca_che_caldo/6790_emergenzacaldo00.html)

- use existing systems and link to general emergency response arrangements;
- adopt a long-term approach (mitigation actions and adaptation of built environment);
- be broad (multi-agency approach);
- communicate effectively;
- ensure that responses to heatwaves do not exacerbate the problem of climate change;
- evaluate (if plans and their implementation are not evaluated, they will not improve).

The World Health Organization identified the following core elements for successful implementation of heat-health action plans (WHO, 2008b):

- agreement of a lead national body;
- accurate and timely alert systems;

- a heat-related health information plan;
- a reduction in indoor heat exposure (medium- and short-term strategies);
- particular care for vulnerable population groups;
- preparedness of the health and social care system;
- long-term urban planning;
- real-time surveillance and evaluation.

Fires

Fire incidents are expected to grow, in particular in the Mediterranean, with increased drought risk. The smoke produced in big vegetation fire incidents, such as those that have occurred in southern Europe, Southeast Asia and other areas, poses not only threats, but also challenges for improving air-quality monitoring in emergency situations, for enhancing personal protection and for developing advanced early warning systems. Coping with all issues of vegetation fire smoke is not a specialized issue; it is both a core disaster discipline and a key methodology that can be applied to other disasters and threats.

Areas of significant interest regarding vegetation fire smoke are: the chemistry of forest fire smoke, medical and toxicological issues of smoke, exposure limits set by international organizations, air-quality monitoring near the flame-front, personal protective equipment, cross-border transfer of smoke and crisis management.

Several pilot projects in relation to fire impact have been developed, aiming to clearly identify high-risk areas, establish effective solutions to control and reduce the spread of fires and to restore affected areas. The MEGAFIRES project, for example, produced a map of fire 'danger' areas in Mediterranean countries, while MEFISTO produced real-time forest fire simulators, and PROMETHEUS studied the effects of fires on vegetation and suggests management methods to limit damage. This information could be made available systematically through health and civil protection systems and also alert hospitals on the potential flow of patients.

Crisis management of forest fire smoke is important because smoke affects not only the population in the vicinity of the fire, but also impacts on populations who live further away from the fire. A number of questions need to be answered:

- Are there any evacuation criteria for coping with short-term health impacts of forest fire smoke?
- Are there any methods or tools for coping with cross-border vegetation fire smoke impacts?
- What are the evacuation procedures?
- Do operational emergency plans include coping with forest fire smoke?
- Is there a need to develop special guidelines and emergency plans for coping with vegetation fire smoke?

Droughts

The provision of sufficient storage capacity for our growing water demands and increasing climate variability is one the main concerns for water managers in the coming decades, requiring careful management of ground water (Tuinhof et al, 2005). Spatial analysis could reveal the degree of threat of progressive drought and related ecological security (Jiao and Xiao, 2004). Analysis of fluctuations in groundwater and the vegetation dependent on it, in relation to each other and wider factors, is important for managing water and predicting vegetation responses (Naumburg et al, 2005).

Virtual water trade has been proposed as a concept to help thinking about water scarcity and management and as a potential solution for water-short countries (Lundqvist and Furuyashiki, 2004). In particular some eastern European countries, the Mediterranean, Africa and Asia will be facing increasing frequency of drought. The biggest impacts are on water shortage – with negative impacts on agriculture with a potential risk of migration. Reuse of waste water and desalinization in coastal areas are among the remedial actions, although these carry some risks related to human health, for example algae and endocrine-disrupting chemicals.

Windstorms

The most common effects on humans from windstorms are road traffic accidents (overturning vehicles, collisions with fallen trees) and individual accidents (being blown over or struck by flying debris/masonry). Building failure represents a less significant, but still important, impact on human life (falling chimneys etc.) (Baker and Lee, 2008). Public health actions are summarized in Figure 12.3.

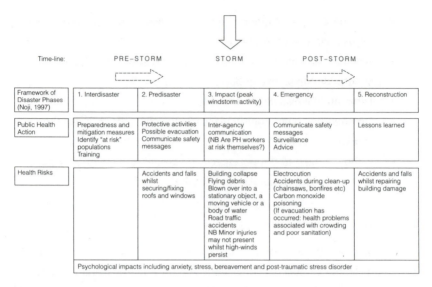

Figure 12.3 Windstorm impacts and related public health actions

Source: Baker and Lee (2008)

Floods

Floods have the greatest damage potential of all natural disasters worldwide and affect the greatest number of people. On a global basis, there is evidence that the number of people affected, and the economic damages resulting from flooding, are rising at an alarming rate. Society must move from the current paradigm of post-disaster response: the current event-disaster cycle must be broken. More than ever, there is the need for decision-makers to adopt holistic approaches for flood disaster management (United Nations, 2004).

Interventions before, during and after floods can reduce short- and long-term health impacts. Hospitals, ambulances, retirement homes, schools and kinder-gartens in flood-prone areas are at risk and the evacuation of patients and vulnerable groups might present a further risk. Crop-growing areas may require specific protection (Casteel et al, 2006). The impact of floods on regional secu-rity, economics, health and political stability is more difficult to measure and quantify. If predictions of increased flooding under future climate change are correct, flooding is an issue that health agencies and civil protection agen-cies have to address by coordinated planning and action and cooperation in preparedness and response.

Specific features of river floods and sea floods have been identified, leading to a range of planning, response and prevention strategies, including non-structural flood-management policies (Poff, 2002). Tsunami risk in Europe should be considered as well and requires specific approaches (Emerson et al, 2005). Health effects can be prevented through a greater emphasis on disaster preparedness and strategies for risk reduction before a flood occurs. This requires a cross-sector approach and includes targeted information to the most vulnerable populations in advance.

Specific lessons learned from flooding events (Briukhanova et al, 2003; Baxter, 2005; Lavery and Donovan, 2005; Brandenburg et al, 2006; Brodie et al, 2006; Buehler et al, 2006; Zoraster, 2006; Beaudoin, 2007; Pitt, 2008) include the need:

- for adequate housing and planning;
- to review all flood risk, including surface water and groundwater;
- to review flood defence and drainage infrastructure;
- to prepare advanced warnings;
- to strengthen social networks to access information;
- to estimate health impacts of structural and non-structural defence mechanisms;
- to prepare and test evacuation plans;
- to establish long-term disease surveillance;
- to review property insurance;
- to modernize flood risk legislation.

Early warning systems

Early warning is the provision of timely and effective information, through identified institutions, that allows individuals exposed to a hazard to take action to avoid or reduce their risk and prepare for effective response (ISDR, 2009). Early warning systems include a chain of actions, namely:

- understanding and mapping the hazard;
- monitoring and forecasting impending events;
- processing and disseminating understandable warnings to political authorities and the population;
- undertaking appropriate and timely actions in response to the warnings.

To be effective, early warning systems for natural hazards need to have not only a sound scientific and technical basis, but also a strong focus on the people exposed to risk. They also need a systems approach that incorporates all of the relevant factors in that risk, whether arising from the natural hazards or social vulnerabilities and from short-term or long-term processes (Basher, 2006).

Public health measures include health promotion and heatwave warning systems (but the effectiveness of acute measures in response to heatwaves has not yet been formally evaluated).

Civil protection and community alerts

With the emphasis on anti-terrorism measures, and a new spirit of authoritarianism, civil defence appears to be becoming resurgent at the expense of the more democratic forms of crisis management inherent in modern civil protection arrangements (Alexander, 2002). Civil defence is a progenitor of civil protection. In an epoch of global terrorism the two must co-exist. The maintenance or restoration of law and order may be fundamental to civil defence, but civil protection is based on the encouragement of social solidarity rather than the repression of antisocial tendencies (Alexander, 2006).

Civil protection requires members of the public to assume progressively more responsibility for their own safety and security. This does not mean abandoning them to their own devices, but ensuring that they understand the risks of disaster and have the means to face up to them. Traditional, indigenous and social coping mechanisms need to be reinforced wherever appropriate (Kirschenbaum, 2004).

Practical actions include community alerts for fragile older persons, development of scenarios when alerts become applicable, buddy systems, liaison arrangements with public agencies, local action groups for upgrading of flooding defences and so on. Technological support may be available (alerts via mobile phone message to carers, satellite networks).

Support for design and evaluation of such community activity may be available through local public health and civil protection departments and could help their development and widespread implementation.

Health systems to support medium- and long-term adaptation

Weather, climate and water influence virtually all human activities, so almost every sector of the economy – health, energy, transport, food security, management of water, tourism – needs meteorological and hydrological services. The World Meteorological Organization (WMO) has issued guidance on how weather-, climate- and water-related information can contribute to the socio-economic development of nations – especially those of the developing world – and the well-being of their populations (WMO, 2004).

Three areas where health practitioners would be able to contribute are: surveillance systems, food and water supplementation systems and adaptation of the built environment. These are described in the following section.

Surveillance systems

Most surveillance efforts have been devoted to infectious diseases. This may not need to change. The advantage of retaining a focus on infections is that the current systems would continue to be used, thereby putting climate-focused surveillance on a solid foundation.

Many new studies have demonstrated significant associations between climate variability and infectious disease transmission (see Chapter 2) and have specifically highlighted the potential for developing climate-based early warning systems. To date, however, only limited experience of full operational applications has been gained. For some diseases, such as malaria and Rift Valley Fever (RVF), early warnings based on climatic conditions are beginning to be used in selected locations to alert ministries of health to the potential for increased risk of outbreaks and to improve epidemic preparedness, but coverage is patchy (Kuhn et al, 2005).

Close collaboration of infectious disease surveillance experts with epidemiologists experienced in climate-related analysis would help to extend, improve and evaluate such systems, in the context of early detection of climate-related trends.

However, a key change for providing surveillance interpretation relevant to climate change adaptation, would be to reframe some of the infectious disease surveillance systems, so that they can be used as elements of a wider 'environmental public health' surveillance framework. A proposed framework for conducting environmental public health surveillance involves data from three points in the process by which an agent in the environment produces an adverse outcome on health status: hazards, exposures and outcomes (Thacker et al, 1996). Within this framework, it would become easier to define and use surveillance systems for the detection of shifts in infectious disease patterns in relation to climatic changes; and public health agencies would be able to recognize the value of existing systems.

Adaptation of the built environment

There are several opportunities to benefit health by addressing climate change, as summarized in Table 12.1 – see also Chapters 4 and 6.

Enhancing food and water security and supplementation

The Food and Agriculture Organization (FAO) defines food security as a 'situation that exists when all people, at all times, have physical, social, and economic access to sufficient, safe, and nutritious food that meets their dietary needs and food preferences for an active and healthy life' (FAO, 2002). As we saw in Chapter 2, the availability, stability, access and utilization of food supplies may be affected as a consequence of climate change (Schmidhuber and Tubiello, 2007).

There is an immense diversity of agricultural practices because of the range of climate and other environmental variables: cultural, institutional and economic factors, and their interactions (Howden et al, 2007). This means there is a correspondingly large array of possible adaptation options. Many defining features of livelihoods on dry lands in Africa and elsewhere can be regarded as adaptive strategies to climate variability (Morton, 2007), for example:

- allocating farm labour across the seasons in ways that follow unpredictable rainfall variations: 'negotiating the rain';
- making use of biodiversity in cultivated crops and wild plants;
- increasing integration of livestock into farming systems;
- working land harder, in terms of labour input per hectare;

Table 12.1 Relationships between the built environment, climate change and health

Built environment category	Link to GHG emissions and climate change	Built environment strategies	Impacts	Health benefits
Transport	Fuel consumption	Increase proportion of people and goods transported by rail rather than roads	Improved air quality	Reduced motor vehicle injuries and fatalities
	Number of vehicle miles travelled per capita	Promote telecommuting	Increased physical activity from walking and cycling	Reduced levels of respiratory illnesses due to improved air quality
	Long distances between homes, jobs, schools and other destinations	Decrease air travel	Enhanced social capital	
		Decrease distances between destinations (denser and mixed use developments)		Reduced likelihood of cardiovascular diseases, some cancers and osteoporosis, due to increased physical activity
	Long distances from farm and factory to market	Increase facilities and opportunities for transit use, walking and cycling		
		Safe routes to school programmes		Improved mental health
		Use of food and goods from local suppliers		
		Infrastructure for alternative fuel generation and distribution		

Built environment category	Link to GHG emissions and climate change	Built environment strategies	Impacts	Health benefits
Buildings	Energy use in: Producing and transporting Construction Heating and cooling Lighting and elevators Building site choice that promotes car dependency and sprawl	Increase use of sustainable, local and/or recycled construction materials and reuse of older buildings Increase heating and cooling efficiency through site orientation, insulated windows, green roofs and natural ventilation Decrease electricity use by occupants by convenient stairs, compact fluorescent bulbs, day lighting, and motion sensor light switches Adopt guidelines for energy-efficient buildings	Improved air quality from reduced coal-generated electricity Increased physical activity from stair use Decreased heat island effects	Reduced levels of respiratory illnesses due to improved air quality Reduced risk of heart diseases, some cancers and osteoporosis due to more physical activity Improved mental health and productivity from use of daylighting Reduced susceptibility to heat-related illnesses

Built environment category	Link to GHG emissions and climate change	Built environment strategies	Impacts	Health benefits
Land use, forestry and agriculture	Deforestation from logging, agriculture and sprawling development	Develop mixed-use communities	Increased physical activity: walking and cycling in mixed-use communities	Reduced likelihood of cardiovascular diseases, some cancers and osteoporosis, due to increased physical activity
		Preserve/expand parks, trails, green space		
	Separation of land uses increases travel	Community gardens and farmers' markets	Improved social capital–parks, trails and contact with nature	Improved mental health
	Buildings constructed in vulnerable areas, such as coastal regions and flood plains	Reduce construction in coastal locations, flood plains and other vulnerable areas	Improved nutrition from locally grown food	Reduced injuries from severe weather events
		Protect, manage and sustain forests		
		Coordinate regional planning		
		Support sustainable logging and agriculture		
		Reduce demand for meat consumption		

Source: Adapted from Younger et al (2008)

- diversifying livelihoods;
- on-farm storage of food and feed;
- late planting of vegetable crops when cereals fail because of drought.

Many planning frameworks for adaptation have been developed in the last decade. It has been suggested that involving stakeholders from project inception is critical to the successful implementation of such frameworks (Howden et al, 2007). Health practitioners could facilitate a participatory approach that would harness scientific knowledge of agricultural systems, while retaining a focus on the values important to stakeholders.

Other possible roles for the health practitioner are in linking physical activity to local opportunities for food growing in gardens and allotments (Transition Town Totnes, 2009); supporting plans for every health organization to minimize wastage at the buying stage; working in partnership with suppliers to lower the carbon impact of all aspects of procurement and promoting sustainable food throughout their business (NHS Sustainable Development Unit, 2009; see also Chapter 11).

Food supplementation systems have been developed largely for areas within developing countries where droughts have caused widespread famine. However, in many countries, including developed ones, the effect of threats to food security may result in increases in food prices. Food supplementation may be required following any disaster, including those linked to climate change.

Fresh water availability is changing in relation to climate warming, as we have seen in Chapters 2 and 3. At the same time, changes in land use are also affecting the availability of water resources. These combined effects have consequences not restricted to estimates of future flood risk, water supply and water quality, but extending to the capacity of engineers to analyse water systems. Therefore, planners will need to adapt the concepts and tools used to analyse water resources, so that water infrastructure, channel modifications and drainage works can be adapted. Such a framework for managing water resources is required urgently, as it is crucial for human adaptation to climate change (Milly et al, 2008).

The temporary suspension of drinking water supply is not uncommon during extreme natural events. Paradoxically, this may occur not only during regular or occasional drought periods, but also during floods. During the 2007 floods in the UK, the affected population lacked access to drinking water for several days and alternative supplies of drinking water were provided by water companies. Public health agencies have a role in setting the minimum amount of drinking water required by categories of individuals in affected populations (Pitt, 2008).

Public health as a function of the local authority (municipality)

The key role of careful energy management in ensuring the transition to sustainable food production, housing and transport has been highlighted (Homer-Dixon, 2007) in this chapter and in Chapter 6. Municipalities need to mitigate *and* adapt, and use the energy available to them in order to achieve integration of these two goals. This requires the prioritization of their efforts and can be summarized as follows (Homer-Dixon, 2007).

Box 12.1
Public health and climate change as a function of the municipality

Municipalities need to act in four areas:

1   overall planning;
2   infrastructure;
3   facilities;
4   emergency preparedness.

Overall planning:

- population density;
- transport;
- vegetation, landscaping;
- disease and pests that affect humans, plants and livestock.

Infrastructure:

- changing risk of unmet water demands; floods; droughts;
- energy;
- sewers.

Facilities:

- schools;
- elderly residential and nursing homes;
- hospitals;
- parks and recreation facilities.

Emergency preparation:

- flood;
- drought;
- heatwaves;
- blackouts.

General advice:

- be creative;
- challenge standard operating procedures;
- work with civil society;
- plan long;
- remember your grandchildren.

Public health competencies for climate adaptation

Public health practitioners are required by academic and government authorities responsible for their education and training to achieve competencies that are relevant to their practice. For example, in the UK the Faculty of Public Health has identified competencies essential for public health practice. The capacity of interpreting and addressing ongoing environmental health issues is often neither described nor supported by the arrangements for education, training and selection of public health practitioners. To achieve the ambitious objectives of adaptation to climate change, an effort to identify and develop relevant climate-related competencies would appear to be required.

To equip the public health workforce with conceptual and practical tools helpful to design adaptations to climate change, a first stage could be the recognition of 'environmental public health', which has been defined as 'the science and art of preventing disease, prolonging life and promoting health where environmental hazards are the key factor, through organized efforts of society' (Spiby, 2006). Examples of competencies relevant for training in environmental public health are:

- understanding the relevance of other agencies and organizations and their roles;
- understanding the principles of ecological sustainability and relevance to public health;
- understanding environmental health policy at international, national, regional and local levels;
- understanding the principles and use of burden of disease methods, health impact assessment and analysis;
- being aware of the main elements of relevant legislation and regulation, e.g. air pollution, land contamination and planning;
- developing and implementing preventive programmes and working towards reducing health inequalities and promoting social inclusion;
- understanding incident planning and incident team management;
- understanding major incident command and control structures;
- understanding the resource implications of environmental incidents, what needs to be paid for and by whom, and the ability to prioritize resource use to ensure cost-effectiveness;
- managing the process, including media skills, risk assessment, communication and analysis.

More specific skills have been identified with regard to adaptation to climate change that would contribute to effective work by health practitioners (Climate Connection, 2009).

Link between evaluation and innovation

Evaluation is a key component of the planning cycle for adaptation. Interventions that have been designed to allow a comprehensive evaluation of social and health impacts, as well as costs and resources required, will provide timely information for the ongoing planning of adaptation strategies.

There is synergy between the effort devoted to designing interventions that are amenable to evaluation and the promotion of innovation in the field of adaptation.

A programme of adaptation that encourages, identifies, supports and highlights innovative adaptation measures is nevertheless desirable. Often an innovative individual may propose an intervention that would traditionally require cycles of selection and testing before being widely applied. This traditional model can be slow and cumbersome and ignore potentially valid and perhaps extremely rewarding interventions. A programme to encourage innovation could be run in parallel with large-scale national evaluations of interventions that are on the point of being implemented in the field.

Action points

The action points offered here focus on adaptation (secondary or tertiary prevention).

1   Do you know the likely local impacts and arrangements for response to extreme weather events (consider floods, droughts, fires heatwaves, cold snaps, landslides and windstorms)?

2   Do you know the contact person in your organization for response to extreme weather events? Ask them for a copy of the local plan.

3   Can you contribute to the development of local plans for response to extreme weather events, in the light of information about the most likely pattern in your area, and your knowledge of the local population who may be vulnerable to the effects?

4   What could be your personal role in preparing and responding to extreme weather events? Consider advice from professional organizations and the World Health Organization (see text and references). Consider your professional contacts with carers and other means of providing health care and social support to those vulnerable to the effects of extreme weather events.

5   Are you able to identify the contact person in your organization or health system for the provision of information to local or national surveillance of infectious disease? Update yourself on agreed arrangements in the light of the changing distribution of vectors and other drivers (see also Chapter 2).

6   What would you do if you identified injuries or other health consequences of extreme weather events? Consider reporting these to a person in your organization or health system interested in this topic, thereby contributing to surveillance programmes.

7   Can you identify people you know, professionally or personally, who may be vulnerable to consequences of a sudden interruption of power supply, such as might occur in the event of an extreme weather event? This might include failure of supply of essential treatment such as oxygen.

8   Can you contribute to the design of 'supply chains' for treatment or equipment, resilient to the possible disruption caused by extreme weather events?

9   Are you familiar with the guidance on possible hardware failures associated with the interruption of power supply or treatments, during and after an extreme weather event?

10 What are your thoughts on longer-term issues such as design of hospitals and health care buildings, in the context of resilience to extreme weather events, and functioning within a low-carbon society?

Please note that the views and opinions presented in this chapter are those of the author and do not necessarily represent the views of the United Kingdom Health Protection Agency.

References

Alexander, D. (2002) 'From civil defence to civil protection – and back again', *Disaster Prevention and Management*, vol 11, no 3, pp209–213

Alexander, D. (2006) 'Symbolic and practical interpretations of the Hurricane Katrina disaster in New Orleans', in 'Understanding Katrina, Perspectives from the Social Sciences', available at: http://understandingkatrina.ssrc.org/Alexander/ (accessed 12 February 2009)

Baker, C. and Lee, B. (2008) 'Guidance on Windstorms for the Public Health Workforce', Health Protection Agency, Chemical Hazards and Poisons Report, Issue 49, September 2008, available at www.hpa.org.uk/web/HPAwebFile/ HPAweb_C/1222068844046 (accessed 11 February 2009)

Basher, R. (2006) 'Global early warning systems for natural hazards: systematic and people-centred', *Philosophical Transactions. Series A, Mathematical, Physical, and Engineering Sciences*, vol 364, pp2167–2182

Baxter, P.J. (2005) 'The east coast big flood, 31 January–1 February 1953: a summary of the human disaster', *Philosophical Transactions. Series A, Mathematical, Physical, and Engineering Sciences*, vol 363, no 1831, pp1293–1312

Beaudoin, C.E. (2007) 'News, social capital and health in the context of Katrina', *Journal of Health Care for the Poor and Underserved*, vol 18, no 2, pp418–430

Brandenburg, M.A., Ogle, M.B., Washington, B.A., Garner, M.J., Watkins, S.A. and Brandenburg, K.L. (2006) '"Operation Child-Safe": a strategy for preventing unintentional pediatric injuries at a Hurricane Katrina evacuee shelter', *Prehospital Disaster Medicine*, vol 21, no 5, pp359–365

Briukhanova, G.D., Grizhebovskii, G.M. and Mezentsev, V.M. (2003) 'Hydrological dangerous natural phenomena as cause of aggravation of an epidemiological situation', *Zhurnal mikrobiologii, epidemiologii, i immunobiologii,* no 6, pp81–86

Brodie, M., Weltzien, E., Altman D., Blendon R.J. and Benson, J.M. (2006) 'Experiences of Hurricane Katrina evacuees in Houston shelters: implications for future planning', *American Journal of Public Health*, vol 96, no 8, pp1402–1408

Buehler, J.W., Whitney, E.A. and Berkelman, R.L. (2006) 'Business and public health collaboration for emergency preparedness in Georgia: a case study', *BMC Public Health*, vol 6, p285

Casteel, M.J., Sobsey, M.D. and Mueller, J.P. (2006) 'Fecal contamination of agricultural soils before and after hurricane-associated flooding in North Carolina', *Journal of Environmental Science and Health. Part A, Toxic/hazardous Substances & Environmental Engineering*, vol 41, no 2, pp173–184

Climate Connection (2009) 'Public Health Competences for Climate Change Mitigation & Resilience', available at www.theclimateconnection.org/public-health-competences-climate-changev3

Ebi, K.L., Smith, J., Burton, I. and Scheraga, J. (2006) 'Some lessons learned from public health on the process of adaptation', *Mitigation and Adaptation Strategies for Global Change*, vol 11, no 3, pp607–620

Ebi, K.L. (2009) 'Public health responses to the risks of climate variability and change in the United States', *Journal of Occupational and Environmental Medicine*, vol 51, no 1

Emerson, N., Pesigan, A., Sarana, L., Motus, N., Buriak, D. and Randall, T. (2005) 'Panel 2.7: first 30 days: organizing rapid responses', *Prehospital and Disaster Medicine*, vol 20, no 6, pp420–422

EU Commission (2007) 'Adapting to climate change in Europe – options for EU action', Green paper from the Commission to the Council, the European Parliament, the European Economic and Social Committee and the Committee of the Regions, SEC(2007) 849}, available at http://ec.europa.eu/environment/climat/adaptation/index_en.htm (accessed 5 December 2008)

FAO (2002) 'The state of food insecurity in the world 2001', Food and Agriculture Organization, Rome

Friel, S., Marmot, M., McMichael, A.J., Kjellstrom, T. and Vågerö, D. (2008) 'Global health equity and climate stabilisation: a common agenda', The Lancet, vol 372, pp1677–1683

Frumkin, H. and McMichael, A.J. (2008) 'Climate change and public health: thinking, communicating, acting', American Journal of Preventative Medicine, vol 35, no 5, pp403–410

Frumkin, H., Hess, J., Luber, G., Malilay, J. and McGeehin, M. (2008) 'Climate change: the public health response', American Journal of Public Health, vol 98, pp435–445, available at www.louisvilleky.gov/NR/rdonlyres/4EB6612D-5274-48AD-9D85-74FBBC3D4860/0/ClimateChangeThePublicHealthResponse.pdf (accessed 12 February 2009)

Homer-Dixon, T. (2007) The Upside of Down: catastrophe, creativity and the renewal of civilisation, souvenir press Ltd, London

Howden, S.M., Soussana, J.F., Tubiello, F.N., Chhetri, N., Dunlop, M. and Meinke, H. (2007) 'Adapting agriculture to climate change', Proceedings of the National Academy of Science, vol 104, no 50, pp19691–19696

ISDR (2005) 'Hyogo Framework for Action 2005–2015', available at www.unisdr.org/eng/hfa/hfa.htm (accessed 18 February 2009)

ISDR (2007) 'Words into Action, a Guide for Implementing the Hyogo Framework for Action 2005–2015: Building the Resilience of Nations and Communities to Disasters', United Nations, available at www.unisdr.org/eng/about_isdr/isdr-publications/02-words-into-action/words-into-action.pdf (accessed 11 June 2009)

ISDR (2008) 'Climate Change and Disaster Risks. ISDR Recommendations for Action Now and Post-Kyoto', available at www.unisdr.org/eng/risk-reduction/climate-change/docs/ISDR%20recommendations%20for%20COP-13.pdf (accessed 11 June 2009)

ISDR (2009) 'Defining a Few Key Terms', available at www.unisdr.org/eng/media-room/facts-sheets/fs-Defining-a-few-key-terms.htm (accessed 11 February 2009)

IPCC (2007) 'Climate Change 2007 – Mitigation of Climate Change', Working Group III contribution to the Fourth Assessment Report of the IPCC, Report of the IPCC, Cambridge University Press

Jiao, Y. and Xiao, D. (2004) 'Spatial neighboring characteristics among patch types in oasis and its ecological security', *Ying Yong Sheng Tai Xue Bao*, vol 15, no 1, pp31–35

Keim, M.E. (2008) 'Building human resilience: the role of public health preparedness and response as an adaptation to climate change', *American Journal of Preventative Medicine*, vol 35, no 5, pp508–516

Kirschenbaum, A. (2004) *Chaos, Organization, and Disaster Management*, Marcel Dekker, New York

Klein, R.J.T., Schipper, E.L. and Dessai, S. (2005) 'Integrating mitigation and adaptation into climate and development policy: three research questions', *Environmental Science and Policy*, vol 8, pp579–588

Klein, R.J.T., Huq, S., Denton, F., Downing, T.E., Richels, R.G., Robinson, J.B. and Toth, F.L. (2007) 'Inter-relationships Between Adaptation and Mitigation. Climate Change 2007: Impacts, Adaptation and Vulnerability', Contribution of Working Group II to the Fourth Assessment Report of the Intergovernmental Panel on Climate Change, Parry, M.L., Canziani, O.F., Palutikof, J.P., van der Linden, P.J. and Hanson, C.E. (eds), Cambridge University Press, Cambridge, UK, pp745–777

Kovats, R.S. and Hajat, S. (2008) 'Heat stress and public health: a critical review', *Annual Review of Public Health*, vol 29, p41

Kuhn, K., Campbell-Lendrum, D., Haines, A. and Cox, J. (2005) 'Using Climate to Predict Infectious Disease Epidemics', World Health Organization, Geneva, available at www.eird.org/isdr-biblio/PDF/Using%20climate%20to%20predict.pdf (accessed 18 February 2009)

Lavery, S. and Donovan, B. (2005) 'Flood risk management in the Thames Estuary looking ahead 100 years', *Philosophical Transactions. Series A Mathematical, Physical and Engineering Sciences*, vol 363, no 1831, pp1455–1474

Lundqvist, J. and Furuyashiki, K. (2004) 'Workshop 7 (synthesis): role and governance implications of virtual water trade', *Water Science and Technology*, vol 49, no 7, pp199–201

McMichael, A.J., Nyong, A. and Corvalan, C. (2008) 'Global environmental change and health: impacts, inequalities, and the health sector', *British Medical Journal*, vol 336, pp191–194

Menne, B. and Ebi, K. (2005) *Climate Change and Adaptation Strategies for Human Health*, Steinkopff Verlag, Darmstadt

Milly, P.C.D., Betancourt, J., Falkenmark, M., Hirsch, R.M., Kundzewicz, Z.W., Lettenmaier D.P. and Stouffer, R.J. (2008) 'Stationarity is dead: whither water management?' *Science*, vol 319, pp573–574

Mitchell, T. and Tanner, T. (2006) 'Adapting to Climate Change: Challenges and Opportunities for the development community', Tearfund, available at www.tearfund.org/webdocs/website/Campaigning/policy%20and%20research/Adapting%20to%20climate%20change%20discussion%20paper.pdf (accessed 18 February 2009)

Morton, J.F. (2007) 'The impact of climate change on smallholder and subsistence agriculture', *Proceedings of the National Academy of Science*, vol 104, no 50, pp19680–19685

Naumburg, E., Mata-Gonzalez, R., Hunter, R.G., McLendon, T. and Martin D.W. (2005) 'Phreatophytic vegetation and groundwater fluctuations: a review of current research and application of ecosystem response modeling with an emphasis on great basin vegetation', *Environmental Management*, vol 35, no 6, pp726–740

NHS Sustainable Development Unit (2009) 'Saving Carbon, Improving Health: NHS Carbon Reduction Strategy for England', available at www.sdu.nhs.uk/page.php?area_id=2 (accessed 11 February 2009)

Noji, E.K. (1997) *The Public Health Consequences of Disasters*, Oxford University Press, New York

Pitt, M. (2008) 'Learning Lessons From the 2007 Floods', UK Cabinet Office, available at http://archive.cabinetoffice.gov.uk/pittreview/thepittreview/final_report.html (accessed 11 February 2009)

Poff, N.L. (2002) 'Ecological response to and management of increased flooding caused by climate change', *Philosophical Transactions. Series A, Mathematical, Physical and Engineering Sciences*, vol 360, no 1796, pp1497–1510

Schmidhuber, J. and Tubiello, F.N. (2007) 'Global food security under climate change', *Proceedings of the National Academy of Science*, vol 104, no 50, pp19703–19708

Semenza, J.C., Hall, D.E., Wilson, D.J., Bontempo, B.D., Sailor, D.J. and George, L.A. (2008) 'Public perception of climate change: voluntary mitigation and barriers to behaviour change', *American Journal of Preventative Medicine*, vol 35, no 5, pp479–487

Spiby, J. (2006) 'Developing competencies in environmental public health', *Chemical Hazards and Poisons Report*, Issue 6, February, available at www.hpa.org.uk/web/HPAwebFile/HPAweb_C/1194947321801 (accessed 18 February 2009)

Stern, N. (2007) *The Economics of Climate Change. The Stern Review*, Cambridge University Press, Cambridge, available at www.hm-treasury.gov.uk/sternreview_index.htm

Thacker, S.B., Stroup, D.F., Parrish, R.G. and Anderson, H.A. (1996) 'Surveillance in environmental public health: issues, systems, and sources', *American Journal of Public Health*, vol 86, no 5, pp633–638

Transition Town Totnes (2009) 'Community Food and Wellbeing Garden', available at www.totnes.transitionnetwork.org/taxonomy/term/116 (accessed 11 February 2009)

Tuinhof, A., Olsthoorn, T., Heederik, J.P. and de Vries, J. (2005) 'Groundwater storage and water security: making better use of our largest reservoir', *Water Science and Technology*, vol 51, no 5, pp141–148

United Nations (2004) 'Guidelines for Reducing Flood Losses', available at www.unisdr.org/eng/library/isdr-publication/flood-guidelines/Guidelines-for-reducing-floods-losses.pdf (accessed 11 February 2009)

WHO (2008a) 'Protecting Health from Climate Change – World Health Day 2008', available at http://www.who.int/world-health-day/toolkit/report_web.pdf (accessed 11 June 2009)

WHO (2008b) 'Heat-health action plans, guidance', Matthies, F., Bickler, G., Cardenosa Marin, N. and Hales, S. (eds), World Health Organization, Regional Office for Europe, available at www.euro.who.int/Document/E91347.pdf (accessed 11 February 2009)

WHO (2009) 'Protecting Health from Climate Change: Global Research Priorities. World Health Organization, available at www.who.int/entity/phe/news/madrid_report_661_final_lowres.pdf (accessed 10 June 2009)

WMO (2004) 'Weather, Climate, Water and Sustainable Development', available at www.eird.org/isdr-biblio/PDF/Weather%20Climate%20Water.pdf (accessed 18 February 2009)

Younger, M., Morrow-Almeida, H.R., Vindigni, S.M. and Dannenberg, A.L. (2008) 'The built environment, climate change, and health: opportunities and co-benefits', *American Journal of Preventive Medicine*, vol 35, no 5, pp517–526

Zoraster, R.M. (2006) 'Barriers to disaster coordination: health sector coordination in Banda Aceh following the South Asia Tsunami', *Prehospital and Disaster Medicine*, vol 21, no 1, s13–18

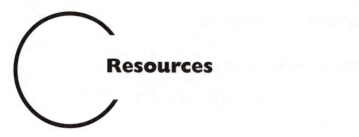

Resources

Organizations and websites

Organizations sponsoring this book

National Heart Forum www.heartforum.org.uk

An alliance of over 60 national organizations in the UK working to reduce the risk of coronary heart disease and associated long-term conditions

National Social Marketing Centre www.nsmcentre.org.uk

A strategic partnership between the Department of Health England and Consumer Focus, working to realize the potential of effective social marketing

United Nations

Intergovernmental Panel on Climate Change www.ipcc.ch

Nobel-prize winning scientific intergovernmental body set up by the World Meteorological Organization and the United Nations Environment Programme to provide decision-makers and others with objective information about climate change. Website has useful graphics, presentations and speeches, as well as IPCC's essential consensus reports

World Health Organization www.who.int/globalchange/climate/en

WHO supports member states in protecting public health from the impacts of climate change, and provides the health-sector voice within the overall UN response to this global challenge; World Health Assembly resolutions, significant publications, speeches by the Director-General

International non-governmental organizations and networks

Climate Action Network Europe www.climnet.org/

Worldwide network of non-governmental organizations and individuals

Friends of the Earth International www.foei.org

The largest grass-roots environmental network, campaigning on today's most urgent environmental and social issues

Health and Environment Alliance (HEAL) www.env-health.org

A network of 60 organizations across Europe, with a track record in increasing public and expert engagement in the EU decision-making process

Health Care without Harm www.noharm.org/

A global coalition, working in more than 50 countries

Medact www.medact.org

A global health charity, led by its health professional membership, campaigning on the health implications of conflict, development and environmental change

WWF www.wwf.org

A global network whose goal is to build a future where people live in harmony with nature

United Kingdom or English organizations

Carbon Trust www.carbontrust.co.uk

Aims to accelerate the move to a low-carbon economy by working with organizations (including the public sector) to reduce carbon emissions

Chartered Institute of Environmental Health www.cieh.org

A professional, awarding and campaigning body for environmental and public health and safety

Climate Connection www.theclimateconnection.org

A public health partnership for action, led by the UK Public Health Association; the UKPHA www.ukpha.org.uk focuses on the need to eliminate health inequalities and promote sustainable development

Climate and Health Council www.climateandhealth.org

Aims to mobilize health professionals across the world to take action to limit climate change

Department for environment, food and rural affairs (Defra) www.defra.gov.uk

UK Government department responsible for sustainable development, whose research, policy and funding initiatives are widely referenced throughout the book

Faculty of Public Health www.fph.org.uk

Works to improve the public's health through education and standards, professional affairs and advocacy and policy

Green Alliance www.green-alliance.org.uk

Aims to make environmental solutions a priority in British politics, working particularly with voluntary sector groups

Health and Sustainable Development Network www.healthandsustainability.net

A network of health practitioners and organizations supporting each other to take action on climate change

Medsin www.medsin.org

A national network of UK students who are interested in global health, part of the International Federation of Medical Students' Association

Natural England www.naturalengland.co.uk

Aims to conserve and enhance the natural environment

NHS Sustainable Development Unit www.sdu.nhs.uk

Develops organizations, people, tools, policy and research to help the National Health Service in England fulfil its potential as a leading sustainable and low-carbon organization

Sustain www.sustainweb.org

Advocates food and agriculture policies and practices that enhance the health and welfare of people and animals; produces publications and guidance

Sustainable Development Commission www.sd-commission.org.uk

The UK Government's independent advisory body on sustainable development; publications and guidance

Sustrans www.sustrans.org.uk

The UK sustainable transport charity, with several important projects, including active travel marketing, and useful publications and guidance

The Met Office www.metoffice.gov.uk/climatechange

Makes substantial contributions to the Intergovernmental Panel on Climate Change and helps inform government policy; practical experience of helping customers to manage the impacts of weather and climate change

Australia

Australian Government Department of Climate Change www.climatechange.gov.au

Wide range of information

Doctors for the Environment Australia www.dea.org.au

Aims to utilize the skills of members of the medical profession to address the ill health resulting from damage to the natural environment, including climate change

India/Asia

India Environment Portal http://indiaenvironmentportal.org.in/

Managed by the Centre for Science and Environment and promoted by the National Knowledge Commission, Government of India; collates and exchanges data, research and information

Tata Energy Research Institute www.terin.org

A non-profit, scientific and policy research organization, working in India and globally in the fields of energy, environment and sustainable development generally

United States of America

Green Guide for Healthcare www.gghc.org

A best practices guide for healthy and sustainable building design, construction and operations for the health care industry

Physicians for Social Responsibility www.psr.org

Works to slow, stop and reverse global warming amongst other aims

Practice Green Health www.practicegreenhealth.org

A membership and networking organization for institutions in the health care community that have made a commitment to sustainable, eco-friendly practices

Publications

Themed issues or series in key journals

American Journal of Preventive Medicine (2008)

Theme Issue: Climate Change and the Health of the Public – 17 papers. Guest Editors: Frumkin, H., McMichael, A.J. and Hess, J.J. Vol 35, no 5, November, www.ajpm-online.net

British Medical Journal (2008)

Vol 336, 28 June: Editor's choice 'Climate change: our new responsibility' by Fiona Godlee; 'Why should doctors be interested in climate change' by M. Gill; 'Ten practical steps for doctors to fight climate change' by J. Griffiths, A. Hill, J. Spiby and R. Stott, www.bmj.com

The Lancet (2007)

Working closely with the London School of Hygiene and Tropical Medicine (including Andy Haines and Ian Roberts), *The Lancet* Series on Energy and Health (six papers and three comments) looks at access to electricity and energy poverty, transport, the built environment, agriculture (including meat consumption), nuclear, and renewable power and other energy issues, and the effect each has on health; it calls for action at all levels; published online, www. thelancet.com/series/energy-and-health

Selected general resources

Chartered Institute of Environmental Health (2008) 'Climate change, public health and health inequalities: a resource for environmental health practitioners', available at www.cieh.org/policy/climate_change_publication.html

Goodall, C. (2007) *How to live a low-carbon life: the individual's guide to stopping climate change*, Earthscan, London, www.earthscan.co.uk/?tabid=318

Griffiths, J. and Stewart, L. (2009) *Sustaining a healthy future: taking action on climate change*, 2nd edition, Faculty of Public Health with the NHS Sustainable Development Unit, NHS Sustainable Development Unit # www.fph.org.uk

Indian National Action Plan on Climate Change, www.pmindia.nic.in/Pg01-52. pdf. Outlines steps to simultaneously advance India's development and climate-related objectives of adaptation and mitigation

UK Public Health Association (2007) 'Climates and change – the urgent need to connect health and sustainable development', www.ukpha.org.uk

Physical activity, active travel and the environment

Department of Health and National Heart Forum (2008) 'Healthy Weight, Healthy Lives: a toolkit for developing local strategies', with the Faculty of Public Health, Department for Children, Schools and Families and Foresight, Government Office for Science, www.dh.gov.uk/en/Publicationsandstatistics/Publications/DH_088968

National Heart Forum, Living Streets and CABE (2007) 'Building health: creating and enhancing places for healthy, active lives: what needs to be done?' National Heart Forum, London, www.heartforum.org.uk/Publications_NHFreports_Pub_BuildHealth.aspx

National Institute for Health and Clinical Excellence (2008) 'Physical activity and the environment', NICE, London, www.nice.org.uk/Guidance/PH8

Managing extreme weather events

Euroheat: publications and tools on how to prevent the adverse health effects of heatwaves, available at www.euro.who.int/globalchange/Topics/20050524_2

Pitt Review: lessons learned from the 2007 floods, reports available at http://archive.cabinetoffice.gov.uk/pittreview/thepittreview/final_report.html

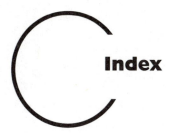

Index